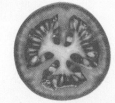

D1031599

Eat Right!

Healthy Eating in College and Beyond

Janet B. Anderson

Nedra K. Christensen

Emily Hoffman

Heidi LeBlanc

Kimberley A. McMahon

Tamara S. Vitale

Meagan Wade

Heidi Wengreen

Utah State University
Nutrition and Food Sciences Department

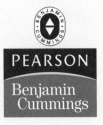

PEARSON

Benjamin
Cummings

San Francisco Boston New York
Cape Town Hong Kong London Madrid Mexico City
Montreal Munich Paris Singapore Sydney Tokyo Toronto

Senior Acquisitions Editor: Deirdre Espinoza
Senior Project Editor: Susan Malloy
Managing Editor, Production: Deborah Cogan
Production Supervisor: Caroline Ayres
Senior Marketing Manager: Sandra Lindelof
Manufacturing Buyer: Stacy Wong

Library of Congress Cataloging-in-Publication Data

Eat right! : healthy eating in college and beyond / Janet B. Anderson ... [et al.].— 1st ed.
    p. cm.
 ISBN 0-8053-8288-7
 1. College students—Nutrition. 2. College students—Health and hygiene. 3. Nutrition. I.
Anderson, Janet B.
 RA777.3.E28 2006
 613.2084'2—dc22

                                                                2005032650

Credits

12 Annie Engel/CORBIS; **7, 12** Brooke Fasani/CORBIS; **80** Bruce James/Getty Images;
22, 25, 34 Burke/Tiolo Productions/Getty Images; **i, iii, v, 4, 5, 6, 19, 20, 23, 28, 38, 40, 41,
44, 45, 46, 47, 52, 70, 72, 73, 86** CORBIS; **48** David C. Ellis/Getty Images; **83** David
Young-Wolff/PhotoEdit; **19, 47, 55, 61, 63, 68, 71** Dorling Kindersley Media Library; **3, 10, 16,
18, 27, 30, 32, 34, 48, 52, 57, 59** Getty Images; **15** Girl Ray/Getty Images; **73** Jack
Anderson/Getty Images; **60** JLP/Jose L. Pelaez/CORBIS; **40** John and Lisa Merrill/CORBIS;
14 Jonathan Kithcen/Getty Images; **37** Joos Mind/Getty Images; **58** Lew Robertson/Getty
Images; **1** Lotus Hoshikawa/Getty Images; **3** Mike/CORBIS; **79** Nathan Bilow/Getty Images;
66 Patrick Giardino/CORBIS; **26** Paul Poplis/Getty Images; **21** Rick Lew/Getty Images;
35, 53, 84, 88 Royalty-Free/CORBIS; **42** Stephen Chernin/Getty Images; **76** Turbo/zefa/CORBIS

ISBN 0-8053-8288-7

10 11 12 13 14 — DOC — 12 11 10 09

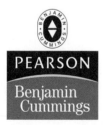

www.aw-bc.com

EAT RIGHT! HEALTHY EATING IN COLLEGE AND BEYOND

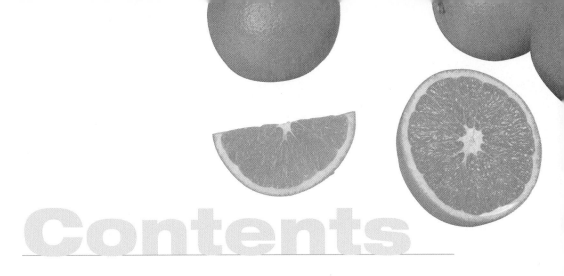

Contents

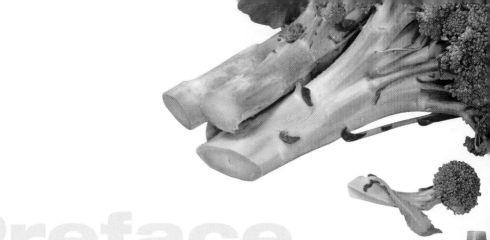

Preface

A century of experience . . . who, us? After adding up our collective years of teaching nutrition to university students and in the community, we found that the grand total came to over 100 years! This number made us cringe and feel ancient, but then the realization came that we're not *that* old, and we do have plenty of experience and wisdom to share with college students.

Through our years as professors, dietitians, and nutrition educators, we have become aware that students are interested in healthy eating, but don't know where to begin. We are excited to be authors of this handbook, and chose topics our students struggle with. The common thread between all chapters is that eating is an enjoyable part of a rich life—not medicine that "should" be taken. Healthy meals for college students can be simple, affordable, *and* delicious.

Students from a variety of majors in a large nutrition course recently did an assignment where they evaluated their own lifestyle and identified one goal, along with their barriers and solutions to that goal. Many students stated that they wanted to improve their diet, and their comments about what they needed to achieve their goals were quite insightful.

- "Cooking classes or food demonstrations that are themed around quick and easy meals."

- "I want to figure out ways to help me change my eating habits now while they are easier to change."

- "I have gotten into a rut and eat only a few different fruits and vegetables. I don't know what is available to purchase or how to use it if I do get it home. Time is a limiting factor."

- "The cost of eating healthy is harder to do on a college budget."

- "Now we are poor, jobless, married college students who can hardly afford the cheap, processed food, let alone healthy, whole grain products."

- "I think planning ahead of time will help instead of hopelessly looking through the cupboards 15 minutes before dinner time."

- "I know that eating processed foods is not the best thing to eat, but it's the lack of time that holds me back from making anything else . . . it's harder to buy food when you are only cooking for one person . . . it will take a lot of work one day, but will pay off in the long run. . . . I would love to start a program at the college that teaches kids like me to cook and stay healthy . . . all of these options will help me and others facing the same issues of going to college and living on our own."

We hope that this handbook will help you with some of these hurdles. It is not meant to provide information "about" nutrition—since you'll get that in your nutrition course! It is meant to be a guide for how to add nutrition to your lives as busy college students, and to help you overcome limits of time, money, or knowledge about how to translate the science of nutrition into the art of food. Our goal is for you to take the information from your nutrition course beyond the final exam, add it to the suggestions in this handbook, and apply it in your cafeteria, grocery carts, and backpacks, and onto your dinner plate.

We sincerely hope that we have provided you with some practical, can-do solutions to eating dilemmas that you can carry with you through life and share with those you love and feed.

This handbook is dedicated to Noreen B. Schvaneveldt, director of Utah State University's Dietetics Programs. She is a wonderful teacher and mentor, well-known for her philosophy of dietary balance: "Never trust a dietitian who doesn't eat ice cream."

Eating Healthy in the Dining Hall

Emily Hoffman

Whether you are trying to lose weight, gain weight, or simply maintain your current weight, eating in the dining hall is often an unhealthy experience. As you start school and get used to dorm life and the dining hall, you may start to wonder whether what you are eating is good for you. Dining halls offer a variety of foods that you can pick from, with no one looking over your shoulder and telling what you should and should not eat. Many students make the mistake of overeating on a daily basis or eating the same food every day because it's their favorite. This chapter will guide you though what a healthy diet is, what foods to focus on, and how to eat healthy in a dining hall or around campus. You'll also get some specifics on picking quick and healthy foods for meals and great snacks to grab and run to class! Let's start by talking about a healthy diet.

What Is a Healthy Diet?

A healthy diet provides the proper combination of energy and nutrients from the foods you eat and has four major elements: adequacy, moderation, balance, and variety.

Adequacy means that your food provides enough energy, nutrients, fiber, and fluids to maintain your health. For example, if you omit meat from your diet and do not replace it with other protein sources, you may become deficient in iron, vitamin B_{12}, and protein, and thus your diet is not adequate.

Moderation means eating the right amounts of food to maintain a healthy weight. If you consume more fat or more calories than your body requires, you will store that excess energy as fat and gain weight.

Balance is eating combinations of foods that provide the proper proportions of nutrients. Michael and Andrew may both need 2,000 kilocalories (kcal) per day total, including 5–7 ounces (oz.) of protein. If Michael eats on average 20 oz. of protein per day, while Andrew eats only 1 oz. of protein per day, neither one is consuming a balanced diet.

Variety comes from eating a lot of different foods each day. For example, men and women ages 19–50 should get 1,000 milligrams (mg) of calcium per day. Milk is not the only source of this nutrient—for variety, you can eat cheese, yogurt, ice cream, spinach, sardines, tofu, and calcium-fortified soy milk.

Why do I need a healthy diet?

A healthy diet helps you maintain or lose weight as needed and gives you more energy for class, sports, and other college activities. A healthy diet can help keep your immune system strong to fight that cold that everyone has in the dorms. It will help you with concentration for taking that big exam, and give you the energy to go to the gym daily or play soccer for the university intramural team. In the long run, a healthy diet will also assist in preventing chronic diseases that usually start affecting you when you are forty years old and older such as heart disease, diabetes, and obesity.

An unhealthy diet is one that lacks any of the components of moderation, variety, balance, and adequacy. For example, you may eat a variety of food that is adequate but lacks moderation and balance, thus leading to an increase in weight and an unhealthy diet. In the short term, poor dietary choices may lead to your being among the 65 percent of American adults considered overweight or obese (National Center for Health Statistics 2004). In the long term, consider that in 2000, several of the leading causes of death were nutrition related, including heart disease, cancer, stroke, and diabetes (Mokdad et al. 2004). An unhealthy diet can lead to serious consequences, while a healthy diet can help keep your body free of chronic and deadly diseases.

What should I eat to stay healthy?

As you put together your healthy diet, remember to aim for *nutrient-dense* foods. Nutrient-dense foods are foods that give you the highest amount of nutrients for the least amount of calories. An example of a nutrient-dense snack is one-half of a whole-wheat bagel with peanut butter, a medium banana, and bottled water, while an example of a non-nutrient-dense snack would be three chocolate chip cookies and a 22 oz. cola.

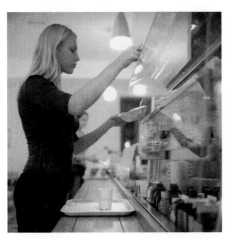
Thinking about your dining hall choices will help you stay healthy.

All food can be part of a healthy diet, but some foods can be consumed more often than others. Fruit needs to be consumed daily, while cookies should be an every-once-in-a-while food. When planning your meals, aim for eating the following foods daily:

Grains—6–11 servings

- Try to make at least half of your grain servings whole grains.
- Eat foods like whole-wheat bread, bagels, pitas, brown rice, whole-grain cereal like oatmeal, and whole-wheat pasta.
- One serving is 1 slice of bread; 1 cup of ready-to-eat cereal; 1/2 cup cooked rice, pasta, or cooked cereal; or 1 handful of whole-wheat crackers.

Fruits—4 servings, or 2 cups

- Try to eat *fresh* fruits as much as possible. They offer more nutrients than canned or frozen fruits and are higher in fiber, which is deficient in many Americans' diets.

- Eat a variety of fruits: try different colors each day (red, purple, orange, yellow, green, and so on).

- Experiment with the many different types of fruits. Try a new fruit like mangos or star fruit.

- One serving is 1/2 cup fruit (fresh, frozen, or canned) or 100% fruit juice, or 1/4 cup dried fruit.

Vegetables—5 servings, or 2 1/2 cups

- The average American does not consume nearly enough vegetables.

- Try to add at least one vegetable to your lunch and dinner, plus at least one snack.

- Make half your plate vegetables (see the "Picture Your Plate" section).

- Vegetables are the perfect food: high in vitamins and minerals, and low in fat and kcals.

- Eat a variety of vegetables; don't stick to just one kind. Every vegetable has different nutrients, and a variety helps keep you healthy.

- One serving is 1/2 cup raw or cooked vegetables or vegetable juice, or 1 cup of raw leafy greens.

Low-fat dairy—3 servings

- Dairy products contain significant amounts of calcium and riboflavin. American diets are typically deficient in these nutrients.

- In addition to dairy products, good sources of calcium include fortified juices and foods, spinach, and tofu.

- One serving is 1 cup milk, 1 1/2 oz. cheese, 1 cup yogurt, 1 cup calcium fortified soy milk, or 1 cup ice cream.

4

Protein—2–3 servings, or 5–7 oz.

- Choose lean meats and prepare them by baking, broiling, and grilling. Avoid fried meats or only eat them occasionally. Go crazy and try some tofu, beans, fish, nuts, and seeds for your protein requirement. You may learn to like some new protein sources (see chapter 5 on vegetarianism for more ideas).

- One serving is 2–3 oz. of meat, poultry, or fish; 1/2 cup cooked dry beans; 2 eggs; 4 tablespoons (tbsp.) peanut butter; or 1 oz. of nuts or seeds.

Healthy fats

- Research points to saturated and trans fatty acids as potentially disease causing, and they should be minimized in our diet.

- While our bodies need some fat, we should focus on polyunsaturated fats (safflower, corn, and soybean oil) and monounsaturated fats (olive and canola oil). Even these healthy fats can be unhealthy if consumed in excess, but a little in our diets can help our heart health and can taste really good too. The next time you make a salad at the salad bar, instead of going for the prepared dressing, drizzle a little olive oil, red wine vinegar, and freshly cracked pepper on it for a true culinary experience!

Empty calories and foods to avoid

- Empty calories are foods that contain a lot of calories but are low in nutrients. They are the opposite of nutrient-dense foods. Empty calories can include sugar-sweetened drinks like soda and juice. Did you know that a 12 oz. can of regular soda contains 9 teaspoons (tsp.) of sugar? That's a lot of sugar. Empty calories can also be the box of cookies in your dorm room or the potato chips in your bag.

- Are these foods okay to eat? Of course they are, as long as you are consuming them less frequently or every once in a while instead of every day. There are more nutrient-dense foods out there to help you maintain your weight and keep your body healthy.

Table 1.1 gives you some more reminders of nutrients that Americans are especially not getting enough of. If you don't consume some of the foods listed, you may not receive enough of these nutrients. You don't need to start buying supplements— just follow the four categories of a healthy diet and be sure to include some of the foods listed so that you can receive all the nutrients needed to stay healthy.

Table 1.1 Are You Missing Out on Nutrients?

If You Don't Eat . . .	You Might Be Missing Out on . . .
Carrots, spinach, sweet potatoes, collards, mixed vegetables, spinach, squash, cantaloupe	Vitamin A
Almonds, fortified cereals, safflower oil, sunflower seeds, mixed nuts, peanut butter, tomato products, avocado, olive oil	Vitamin E
Cheese, milk, soy milk, tofu, yogurt, calcium-fortified products, spinach	Calcium
Bran cereal, fish, pumpkin, spinach, squash, nuts, beans, tofu, whole grains	Magnesium
Fish, potatoes, sweet potatoes, tomato products, white beans, yogurt, peaches, spinach	Potassium
Beans, bran, fruits, lentils, vegetables, whole grains	Fiber

Making the Most of Your Dining Hall

Eight quick tips to jumpstart dining hall health

1. Always eat breakfast.

Eating breakfast has been connected with weight loss and maintenance. In one study, three-fourths of individuals who had lost weight and maintained that weight loss reported eating breakfast daily (Wing and Phelan 2005). In the NHANES study, a large-scale study across the United States, individuals who ate cereal and cooked cereal had lower body mass indexes (BMIs) than people who skipped breakfast (Cho et al. 2003). Eating breakfast can also jumpstart your day by providing essential carbohydrates and protein to get you going and keep you from being hungry during class or at the gym.

2. Focus on fruits and vegetables.

Fruits and vegetables are low in fat and calories and high in fiber. Always include at least one for each of your meals and snacks.

3. Drink milk at meals.

One of the easiest ways to get your calcium is to drink milk or calcium-fortified soy milk with meals. It is easy to remember, will stop soda temptations, and will be habit forming!

4. Follow your hunger cues.

Learn to listen to your body. Make sure you always feel hungry before you eat; otherwise, you may be storing that excess energy as fat! You don't have to be starving, but always ask yourself: am I hungry? Would a cold glass of water help? Or maybe a piece of fruit instead of a cheeseburger and onion rings?

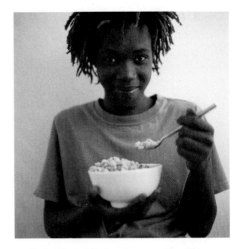

Eating breakfast gets your day off to a great start.

5. Avoid seconds and thirds.

Many dining halls are all-you-can-eat, which means you can go back as many times as necessary until you are stuffed! Try this instead: after you eat your first plate of food, wait at least fifteen minutes before you go back to get seconds. Give yourself time to feel full (sometimes it takes longer than fifteen minutes to feel full). If you are still hungry after dinner, skip the dessert table and get a piece of fruit to dip in yogurt, or some nonfat frozen yogurt topped with fresh peaches or strawberries.

6. Look for whole grains.

Whole grains are good for you! They contain extra fiber and they make you feel fuller than white refined grains do. Look for products that say *whole wheat* or *whole grains*. Try some hot oatmeal one cool morning, use brown rice with your stir-fry, make a sandwich loaded with vegetables on whole-wheat bread, or choose whole-wheat pasta for your dinner (ask your dining hall manager to switch).

7. Schedule your meal times.

Scheduled meal times may sound a little odd, but it helps you establish a pattern. If you follow that pattern, it will help you eat before you are overhungry, which usually leads you to eat anything and everything in sight. Scheduled meal times can also help you plan out what you are going to eat and how to make some healthy choices. It also helps you anticipate the need for snacks or quick meals if you are going to be on the run for most of the day (see the "Doing the Dining Hall Dash" section).

8. Remember 90–10.

And finally, follow the 90–10 rule: eat healthy 90% of the time, eat what you want 10% of the time!

Picture your plate

A quick and easy way to see if you are eating the right portions of foods is to use your plate as your guide. One-half of your plate should always be vegetables or fruits, depending on the meal and what you have planned. One-fourth should be protein, and the other fourth should be whole grains. Pay attention to serving sizes and remember, you don't need to supersize your plate!

Some other plates that add up to a healthy meal:

Breakfast
- Oatmeal with fresh strawberries and blueberries, with milk
- Scrambled eggs with ham, whole-wheat toast, and fresh fruit salad, with milk

Lunch
- Baked potato with cottage cheese and salsa, whole-wheat roll, and apple slices, with milk
- Veggie ham sandwich with cucumber and tomato salad, with milk

Dinner
- Pasta with marinara sauce, broccoli, and apple for dessert, with milk
- One slice pizza with salad and steamed green beans, with milk

Making better choices around the dining hall

At the cold cereal bar	Choose whole-grain cereals.
	Look for 2 grams (g) or more of fiber per serving.
	Always use skim or 1% milk to keep fat content down.
	Try these cereals:
	Cheerios, Bran flakes (Raisin Bran), Wheat Chex, Banana Nut Crunch, Post Blueberry Morning, Wheaties, Frosted Mini-wheats,

Grape-nuts, Quaker Life Cereal, Quaker Oatmeal Squares, Total, any multigrain cereal, and low-fat granola.

At the salad bar	Always go for a darker lettuce, which has more nutrients. Try romaine, red leaf or green leaf lettuce, and other mixes.
	Mix some spinach (which is packed with nutrients) into your lettuce.
	Go for other vegetables such as tomatoes, carrots, cucumbers, peas, beets, radishes, onions, unsalted sunflower seeds, nuts, mushrooms, beans (for example, chickpeas [garbanzo beans] or kidney beans), broccoli, cauliflower, peppers, celery, and corn.
	Add dried fruit (cranberries or other options).
	Go for a low-fat or fat-free dressing, or try drizzling on olive oil and balsamic or red wine vinegar for a tasty treat.
	Items to stay away from include lots of cheese, full-fat cream dressings (ranch and Thousand Island), bacon bits, or anything fried (such as chicken wings or onion rings).
	How to get protein: add a hard-boiled egg, some grilled chicken strips, or cottage cheese, or sprinkle some chickpeas and kidney beans on your salad.
At the grill	Most items on the grill menu aren't everyday choices, but in moderation they can fit into a healthy diet.

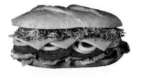

If you want chicken strips or a cheese-burger for dinner, skip the fries. Go for baked chips (Sun Chips or Baked Lays) or a veggie-packed side salad with fat-free dressing instead.

If you want fries, plan ahead and eat a low-fat breakfast and lunch.

If you order sandwiches from the grill, always load up sandwiches with healthy vegetables (lettuce, tomatoes, onions, and peppers).

At the pasta bar

Choose red sauces instead of white sauces. Marinara sauce is usually much lower in calories and fat compared to the Alfredo sauce.

Remember that one serving of pasta is a half cup. You can get away with eating 1 cup of pasta, but don't go overboard with your servings. Remember that half your plate should be vegetables!

Add some cooked vegetables like zuc-chini, summer squash, broccoli, cauli-flower, and carrots to your pasta sauce and create a pasta primavera your friends will envy.

Top off your pasta bar with a whole-wheat roll or breadstick, a salad, or steamed vegetables.

Making the right choices

Now that you can see the options you have at the dining hall, let's compare one day's worth of dining choices to see if we can maximize our healthy diets. In Table 1.2, we've compared two versions of breakfast, lunch, and dinner. Both are a full day's worth of meals, but the healthy choices menu is one-third the fat

Table 1.2 Healthy Choices Add Up in the Dining Hall

	Healthy Choices	Could Be Better
Breakfast	1 cup Honey Nut Cheerios 1 cup skim milk 1/4 cup blueberries 3/4 cup cantaloupe 1 hard-boiled egg 1 cup coffee	1 medium doughnut 1 cup latte

Lunch	Grilled chicken salad:
	2 cups lettuce and assorted
	   vegetables
	3 oz. grilled chicken strips
	
	2 tbsp. fat-free Italian salad
	   dressing
	Whole-wheat roll
	1 tbsp. butter
	1 cup skim milk
		1/4-pound cheeseburger
		1 medium french fries
		
		Bottled water

Snack	1/2 whole-wheat bagel 2 tbsp. light cream cheese Orange 12 oz. diet soda	22 oz. soda Snickers candy bar
Dinner	3 oz. teriyaki chicken 1/2 cup brown rice 1/2 cup fresh or canned pineapple 1/2 cup steamed mixed vegetables 1 tbsp. butter	3 oz. fried chicken 1/2 cup broccoli 1 white roll 1 baked potato 3 tbsp. butter
Snack	2 cups light popcorn 1 cup Orange Julius	No snack
Total kcal Total fat (g) Total protein (g)	1,852 51 108	2,880 154 84

and 1,000 calories less than the unhealthy choices. It also provides a more significant amount of the protein you need every day.

Doing the dining hall dash

Getting healthy food on the go can be tricky, but here are a few options when you are on the run and need something fast from the dining hall or convenience store:

Single foods

- Whole fruit—nature's perfect packaging! (Try apples, oranges, bananas, and blueberries.)

- 1% or skim milk, or 1% chocolate milk—with all those nutrients and protein, it packs a powerful punch.

- Yogurt or yogurt smoothies—watch the fat content. On some smoothies, it may be higher than you expect.

- Trail mix—try mixing low-fat granola, dried cranberries, almonds, peanuts, and dark chocolate chips.

- Almonds—you only need a handful to give you some good fat and protein.

- Pistachios.

- String cheese.

- Whole-wheat crackers.

- Healthy cereal—good to munch on when you are in class.

- Grab-and-go sandwich made from whole-wheat bread.

- Vegetarian wrap.

- Granola bars.

- Low-fat popcorn—try the new mini-bags so you don't overeat.

- Dried fruit.

- Bottled water.

- Prepackaged, cut-up fruit.

Perfect combinations

- Peanut butter with crackers, a bagel, or apples and celery

- Baby carrots, pretzels, and hummus

- Cottage cheese and fruit, vegetables, and/or whole-wheat crackers

- Strawberries with dark chocolate

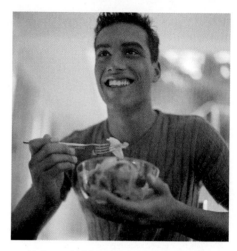

At the salad bar, add a variety of vegetables and proteins such as beans or cheese.

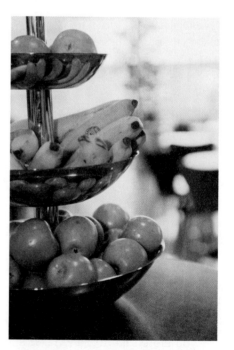

Fruit is a great "grab-and-go" snack.

12

- String cheese, whole-wheat crackers, and a piece of fruit
- Grab-and-go sandwich and a piece of fruit
- Yogurt with breakfast cereal sprinkled on top

Taking action in your dining hall

Have you noticed that there are certain foods lacking in the dining hall (soy milk, skim milk, or fresh fruits and vegetables) or certain healthy foods that run out fast? There are many ways in which you can initiate change in your dining hall. The easiest way is to contact the dining hall manager or the food service director. An in-person visit, or a letter or e-mail, may be enough to make the change you have in mind. Suggestion boxes may also be posted around the dining hall if you don't feel comfortable speaking directly to the manager.

Many dining halls have a student menu committee. Being on such a committee is a great experience and can help bring about the changes you think would enhance the dining hall. You can help plan special events, bring in new foods, or be part of taste panels. You may be asked to help with menu planning, ideas for theme nights, and many other activities.

Make other students aware of healthy foods. Remember, if enough students want a particular food item, the dining hall will find a way to get it. Supply and demand works in dining halls!

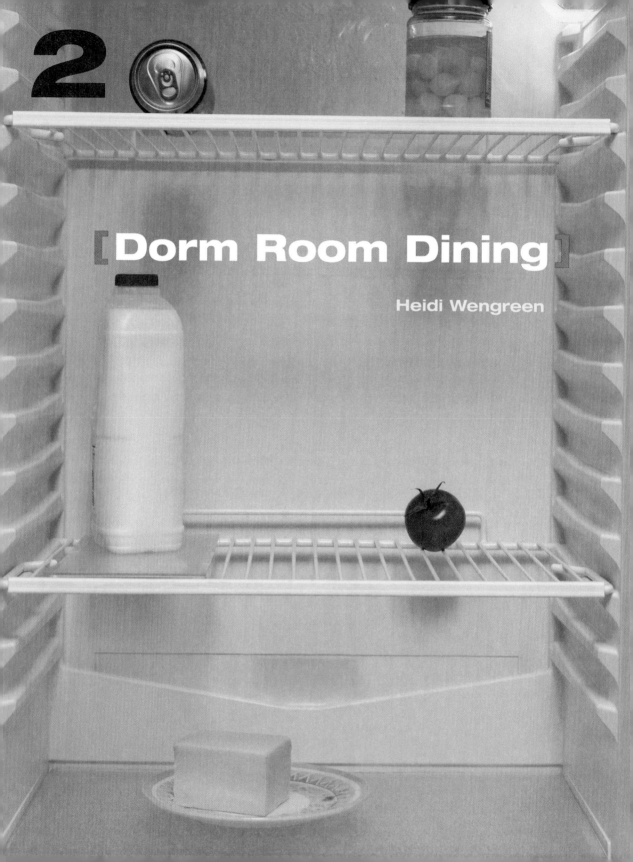

[Dorm Room Dining]

Heidi Wengreen

If you live in on-campus housing and rely on a meal plan, you'll soon find out that eating in the dining hall is not always convenient or appealing. The dining hall isn't available 24/7, you can't wander in for a late-night study snack, you can't dine in private, and you don't have much control over what and when you eat. If you choose wisely, grab-and-go snacks and meals prepared in your dorm room can be a valuable part of a healthy diet. Given the physical restraints of the typical college dorm room, this may seem like a challenge, but with the guidelines and practical tips presented here, you'll be on your way to eating well in your dorm room.

Keys to Eating Well in Your Dorm Room

1. **Plan ahead.** Know the equipment you need and how to prepare your food safely. Make a list before you go shopping, so you choose a variety of foods that you will be able to use. Keep a variety of tasty, nutritious, ready-to-eat foods on hand ready to eat in your room or to take with you when you know you'll be away for more than three hours. This will save you from impulse eating at vending machines and convenience stores where making good nutritious choices is even more of a challenge.

2. **Choose snacks and meals with balance, moderation, and variety in mind.** Snacks that are planned, balanced, and small help fuel your body and brain with the nutrients needed to sustain activities throughout your day. Be sure the snacks and meals you prepare contain lower-fat options from at least two of the five major food groups (whole grains, fruit, vegetable, milk and dairy, and meat and protein). This will help ensure that you are getting a balanced mix of all of the vitamins and minerals found in healthy foods.

3. **Don't skip meals—especially breakfast.** You've heard it a million times: breakfast is the most important meal of the day. But did you know that eating breakfast could actually help improve your grades?

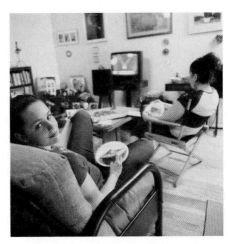

Eating in your dorm room gives you an alternative to the dining hall, but you have many options beyond pizza delivery.

4. Eat when you are hungry—but not for other reasons. Don't get into the habit of eating in your room when you are bored, frustrated, or stressed. This can add extra calories that contribute to weight gain. A better idea is to deal with these feelings in other ways. Take a study break, go for a walk, or call a friend!

Plan Ahead

Have the right equipment

You probably won't be preparing seven-course gourmet meals from your dorm room, but with a little planning there are many options for preparing simple and healthy foods. The first step is to acquire a few pieces of essential equipment. Check with your school's Student Housing Office to see what is allowed and what is not allowed at your particular school. A small microwave and mini-refrigerator are must-haves and are normally allowed in dorms. Arrange with your roommate beforehand to decide who will bring what. You will only need one microwave and other small appliances, but you may both want your own refrigerator. Other appliances that are nice to have if permitted are a coffee maker, blender, and rice cooker. Usually anything with an exposed heat coil, like a hot plate or toaster oven, is off limits.

In addition to appliances, you will need the following:

- Microwave-safe dishes including a medium-sized bowl, a small bowl, a plate, and a cup
- Microwave-safe measuring cup in a pint size
- A handheld can opener
- A large Tupperware-type container to wash dishes in if you don't have a sink
- Dish soap
- Dish towels
- Paper towels

- Utensils
- Pot holder
- Plastic or wire crates to store dry goods and tools
- Knife
- Cutting board
- Antibacterial kitchen cleaning solution
- Sealable sandwich bags
- Paper cups

Be safe: Fires and food-borne illnesses

Cooking is the second leading cause of dorm fires (after arson) and the leading cause of fire injuries, according to the National Fire Protection Association. When you are cooking, stay focused on cooking. Most cooking fires start because of inattentiveness, and most burns or other injuries occur because of carelessness. Always use a pot holder when removing anything from the microwave to prevent burns, and use care when handling knives.

Unlike meals at the dining hall, when you are preparing your own food, the responsibility for food safety is up to you. Health experts estimate that millions of cases of food-borne illness occur in the United States each year, although many cases go unreported because the symptoms are mistaken for the flu or a cold. These symptoms include fatigue, chills, fever, dizziness, headaches, upset stomach, diarrhea, and stomach cramps.

The cause of most cases of food-borne illness is improper food handling, which results in bacterial contamination of prepared foods. Three simple rules can help prevent food-borne illnesses:

1. **Keep food and food preparation areas clean.** This includes your hands. When preparing food, wash your hands frequently, especially after handling raw food. Use clean towels, cooking dishes, knives, and utensils. Be sure to sanitize cutting boards and other food preparation surfaces, and let them air dry after washing.

2. **Keep hot food hot.** High temperatures kill most bacteria. Cooked foods including meat, poultry, fish, and eggs should be cooked to a temperature higher than 140°F and should never be allowed to sit at room temperature for longer than two hours.

3. **Keep cold foods cold.** If cooked foods are to be eaten cold, rapidly cool the food and store it in the refrigerator. In addition to cooked foods, milk and dairy products including yogurt and cheese need to be stored in the refrigerator. You can cool hot food by placing it in a sealable plastic container or baggie and running cold water over it until it is cool.

Make a shopping list

Once you have the essential equipment and understand how to stay safe while cooking, the next step is to go shopping. You will want to keep a good supply of both perishable and nonperishable food staples on hand from which you can prepare a good variety of meals and snacks. Of course, the foods that you choose will be largely determined by your likes, dislikes, and the amount of space you have to store them.

Some ideas for your shopping list:

Grab-and-go ingredients

- Cheese—Cheese in general is a higher-fat food but is a good source of protein and calcium. Choose white cheese over yellow cheese for a lower-fat option. String cheese is a great "grab-and-go" option.

- Yogurt—Pint-sized containers can save you money over single-serving containers but single-serving containers are a good "grab-and-go" option. Choose low-fat varieties.

- Fresh fruit such as apples, oranges, bananas, grapes, or whatever you like—Buy only a couple of pieces of each variety so they don't spoil before you eat them.

- Fresh vegetables—Precut and washed baby carrots are an easy item to cook in the microwave or are a great "grab-and-go" option.

- Nuts—Use your favorites in a trail mix with granola and dried fruit. Nuts are generally a great source of essential fatty acids.

- Dried fruits—Buying from bulk bins is cheaper than individual packages. Toss it with nuts and granola for a great "stash-and-dash" snack.

- Granola—Surprisingly granola is often high in fat, so look for a lower-fat option. Granola makes a great snack when eaten with nuts and dried fruit.

- Pretzels—Pretzels are a lower-fat snack option than chips.

Meal builders

- Eggs—Eggs can be easily poached or scrambled in the microwave and are a good source of protein.

- Cottage cheese—Great by itself, topped with fruit, or mixed with a flavoring as a dip for veggies or crackers.

- Frozen vegetables—These can be easily cooked in the microwave and eaten with rice and pasta or added to soups.

- Sandwich bread, pita bread, and tortillas—Whole-wheat varieties are a better option than white varieties.

- Canned vegetables—This is another way of keeping vegetables on hand. Look for lower-sodium varieties.

- Canned fruits—If you are worried about fresh food going bad, try some canned choices. Be sure it is in its own juice, not syrup.

continued

- Canned meats—Canned tuna, chicken, and shrimp don't need to be refrigerated until after they have been opened, and they are a great source of protein. Use them to make sandwiches or add some to pasta or rice for a quick meal.

- Canned beans—Canned kidney, black, chili, or refried beans are great and cheap sources of fiber and protein. They can easily be added to soups and rice or pasta dishes.

- Canned soups—Look for lower-sodium varieties.

- Salsa and tomato sauce—Tomato-based sauces are full of important antioxidants and when added to rice or pasta make a quick meal.

- Cold cereal—Look for options where a whole grain is the first ingredient. Many cold cereals are fortified with vitamins and minerals like folate and iron.

- Peanut butter—This old stand-by is actually a good source of protein and healthy forms of fat. Look for brands with the least added sugars.

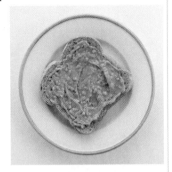

Peanut butter is easy to keep on hand and is full of protein.

Other essentials

- Salt, pepper, and your favorite spices and seasonings—A little spice can go a long way in making food taste better.

- Onion soup mixes or other dry flavoring mixes—Stirred into cottage cheese, these can be used to create healthy dips for vegetables, pretzels, or crackers.

Focus on Balance, Variety, and Moderation

Snack strategies

No food or beverage contains all of the nutrients that a body needs. This means that to get all of the nutrients your body needs from foods, you need to consume a variety of different foods every day, whether it's in your dorm room, dining hall, or elsewhere. It's very easy to fall into a food "rut"—especially when you are on a tight schedule and a tight budget—but eating the same things every day will probably leave you with nutritional holes. For example, carrots are a great source of beta-carotene but they provide little folate and calcium. If the only vegetable you eat is carrots, you will miss out on other important nutrients. Other

Table 2.1 How Do Snacks Contribute to a Healthy Diet?

Snack	% Provided of Daily Nutrient Need*
1 cup yogurt	25% of calcium
1 banana	33% of vitamin B_6, 12% of potassium
10 baby carrots	> 100% of vitamin A
1 medium orange	> 100% of vitamin C
1 cup cottage cheese	50% of protein, 30% of calcium
1/2 cup salsa	10% of potassium, 20% of vitamin C
1 oz. string cheese	25% of calcium
Handful of nuts and dried fruit	100% of biotin, 22% of magnesium
1 cup of broccoli and cauliflower flowerettes	21% of vitamin A
3/4 cup tomato juice	50% of vitamin C

*Based on daily values for a 2,000 calorie per day diet.

vegetables like spinach and broccoli are good sources of folate and calcium but poor sources of beta-carotene. If you have a variety of foods available to snack on, you're likely to have a better balanced diet. Table 2.1 shows how many grab-and-go snacks can be a part of a balanced diet.

An easy way to get extra nutritional benefits from each snack you eat is to be sure each one includes foods from at least two different food groups. Try these ideas for great two food-group snacks:

1. Whole-grain fortified cereal and 1 cup milk
2. Apple wedges and a mozzarella cheese stick
3. 3 cups popcorn sprinkled with 2 tbsp. parmesan cheese
4. 10 pretzels, 1 ounce of cheese, and mustard
5. Microwave cheese quesadilla (tortilla, 1/4 cup shredded cheese, and 1/4 cup salsa)
6. 2 tablespoons hummus and half a pita pocket in slices
7. 1 cup yogurt and nuts or dried fruit

8. Trail mix (granola, nuts, and dried fruit)

9. Cottage cheese and fruit (canned mandarin oranges or peaches)

10. Fruit smoothie (fruit, fruit juice, milk, and yogurt blended together)

Most of these snacks can be adapted to be "stash-and-dash" so that they can be prepared beforehand, packed with you when you leave, and eaten later in the day. For example, fruit parfaits can be made in disposable paper cups and taken with you as you dash out the door in the morning for breakfast. Peanut butter, hummus, or cottage cheese for dipping fruit, vegetables, or crackers can be stored in a small paper cup enclosed in a sandwich bag.

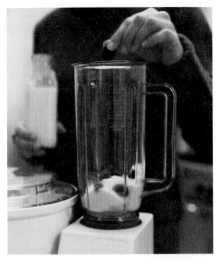

Smoothies are an easy way to add fruit and dairy to your diet.

If you're on the go and want to keep cold snacks cold, stash a water bottle in your freezer before you go to bed. In the morning, pack your snacks with your frozen water bottle in a small, insulated lunch bag. The frozen water bottle will keep your snacks cool during the day and will eventually melt and be ready for drinking. (Health experts generally recommend that you drink about 8 cups, or 64 fluid ounces, of water every day.)

Microwave it

Microwaves aren't just for popping popcorn or heating up water. Try these ten healthy and hot meal ideas you can cook up in a microwave.

1. **Canned soup**—Add beans, canned meat, pasta, or vegetables to basic soups.

2. **Bean burrito**—Spread refried or black beans on a tortilla, sprinkle with shredded cheese, roll up, and microwave for forty-five seconds.

3. **Quesadilla**—Spread refried or black beans on a tortilla, sprinkle with shredded cheese, microwave for thirty seconds, cut into triangles, and dip in salsa.

4. **Veggie burgers**—Burgers made from soy protein and vegetables can be found in the frozen food section of your local supermarket. Heat according to the package directions. Eat on a bun with your favorite burger toppings.

5. **Vegetable stir-fry**—Put frozen or fresh sliced or diced vegetables in a bowl and microwave for about four minutes. Add your favorite seasoning, sauce, or canned shrimp or chicken. Serve over rice or pasta, or wrap in a pita pocket or tortilla.

6. **Scrambled eggs**—Beat two eggs in a bowl, then add 2 tbsp. of milk, and salt and pepper. Pour eggs into microwave safe bowl and microwave for 3–4 minutes. Add cheese, or vegetables such as chopped tomatoes, broccoli, or mushrooms.

7. **Smothered potato**—Microwave a potato on high for ten minutes. Top with shredded cheese and canned chili.

8. **Mini-pizza**—Top English muffins, bagels, or pita pockets with tomato sauce, a dash of oregano and garlic powder, and then shredded cheese. Microwave for one minute. Be creative with additional toppings like diced green peppers, olives, and pineapple.

9. **Frozen entrée**—If you choose options that are lower in fat, simple sugars, and sodium, frozen dinners can be a fast and nutritious option. Heat according to the package directions.

10. **Pasta with sauce and vegetables**—Add 1 1/2 quarts of water and 1/2 tsp. salt to a 2-quart microwave-safe casserole dish. Cook on high 3–4 minutes until water boils. Add 1 cup small noodles (shells, macaroni, rotini) and cook for twelve minutes on low power. Drain water from dish, and add your favorite sauce and vegetables. Cook an additional thirty seconds.

No cooking needed

There are healthy snacks and meals you can make without any cooking at all. Try sandwiches made from peanut butter and banana or apple slices; cold cereal and milk topped with fruit; pita pocket sandwiches made from canned tuna or chicken, a tablespoon of salad dressing, and tomato slices; and yogurt parfaits of yogurt, granola, fruit, and nuts. For the healthiest versions of these meals, choose low-fat yogurt, whole-wheat bread, tuna packed in water, and reduced-fat salad dressing. In addition, include a fresh fruit and vegetable in your no-cook meal. A tuna salad pita pocket with an apple and carrot sticks on the side is a very balanced and nutritious no-cook meal.

Prepackaged choices

Frozen entrées and prepackaged foods are another alternative for dorm-room dining. Use labels to compare prepackaged foods at the grocery store. Although they are convenient and fast, these foods often contain more of the ingredients we try to avoid, like trans fats and sodium, than their home-prepared versions. Be sure to check the serving size: the "Nutrition Facts" section of the label lists amounts per serving of the food, but serving sizes for similar foods may differ. Look for options that provide less total fat, saturated fat, trans fats, cholesterol, sodium, and sugar per serving and more dietary fiber, protein, vitamin A, calcium, vitamin C, and iron per serving.

Also look at the "% Daily Values" section for a general idea of how one serving of the food contributes nutritionally to a 2,000 calories a day diet. Daily values can be used as a guide to see if a food provides a little or a lot of a given nutrient. The ingredient list is also a helpful indicator as ingredients must be listed in order from most to least. For example, stay away from cereals where sugar or high-fructose corn syrup is listed as the first ingredient. A better choice is a cereal that lists whole-grain wheat as the first ingredient.

A day of healthy dorm room dining

It's very possible to eat an entire day's worth of healthy snacks and foods prepared and cooked from your dorm room. Table 2.2 gives one example of a day of dorm room eating.

Table 2.2 A Day of Healthy Dorm Room Dining	
Time	Food
7 a.m.	Yogurt parfait—1 cup low-fat yogurt, 3 tablespoons mixed nuts and dried fruit, and 1/4 cup granola
10:30	1 medium apple and a 1.5 oz. cheese stick
12:30 p.m.	2 tablespoons peanut butter and 1 medium banana in a whole-wheat tortilla 10 baby carrots Small bunch of grapes
3:00	1/2 cup trail mix 6 oz. boxed fruit drink
6:30	1 cup brown rice 1 cup mixed vegetables *continued*

	1/4 cup canned chicken 3/4 cup mandarin oranges 1 cup low-fat chocolate milk
9:00	1/2 bag low-fat microwave popcorn with cayenne pepper and 2 tablespoons parmesan cheese

Nutrition facts: 2,220 kcalories, 94 grams of protein, 412 grams of carbohydrate, 72 grams of fat, and > 100% DV of vitamin A, thiamin, riboflavin, niacin, vitamin B_6, vitamin B_{12}, vitamin C, biotin, calcium, magnesium, and potassium

Don't Skip Meals, Especially Breakfast

Breakfast is the most frequently omitted meal and is especially easy to skip when a tight schedule requires you to be in class by 7:30 a.m. Studies show that those who regularly eat breakfast perform better in school and score higher on tests of memory and cognition than those who don't eat breakfast.

Try these two-minute grab-and-go breakfast ideas:

1. **Yogurt parfait**—Your favorite low-fat yogurt in a paper cup topped with lower-fat granola, nuts, and fresh or dried fruit.

2. **Peanut butter and banana tortilla**—Spread 1 tbsp. of peanut butter on a tortilla, and roll it up around a peeled banana.

3. **Cold cereal, trail mix, and milk**—Toss your favorite whole-grain cold cereal with nuts and dried fruit. Wash it down with a cold glass of milk.

4. **Instant breakfast beverage**—These are a bit pricey at the store but are a great way to get in a nutritious breakfast. Many varieties provide a good dose of many vitamins and minerals. When mixed with milk, they are also a good source of protein and calcium.

5. **Instant oatmeal**—Sprinkle with your favorite fruit for extra flavor and nutrition.

3

Fast Foods

From Frenzy to Friendly

Nedra K. Christensen

Heidi LeBlanc

Meagan Wade

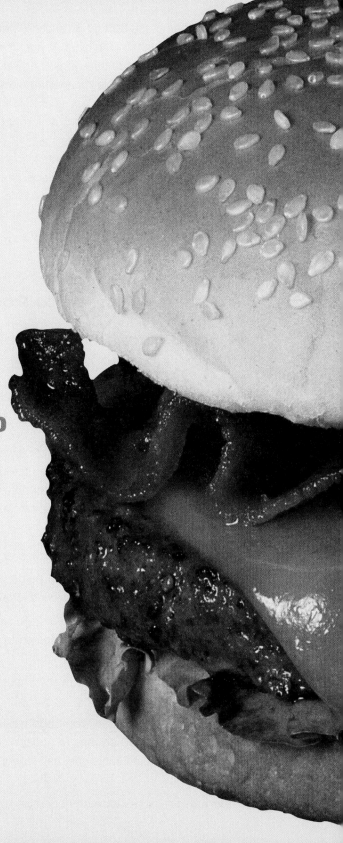

Are you one of the 30% of Americans who ate in a fast food restaurant today? Did you know that by the eighth grade, more than 25% of children eat at a fast food restaurant two to three times per week? Consider that French fries are the most common vegetable in children's diets by the age of eighteen months, and only 67% of two year olds get any fruit in their diet on a given day. Are such eating patterns related to the epidemic of childhood obesity? These habits start early and can continue for a lifetime.

Eating frequently at restaurants (especially fast food restaurants), where you do not have control of the ingredients and cooking techniques used, can have a negative effect on your long-term eating habits, waistline, and general health. Understanding how to control portions at fast food restaurants and how to make healthy choices from the options you encounter will help make fast food a friendly experience, not a frenzy.

Paying Attention to Portion Sizes

Food portions have been supersized

Would you guess that food portion sizes have increased, stayed the same, or decreased in size in recent years? The American Cancer Institute commissioned a survey in 1999 (called the "eyeball method" survey) to raise awareness of how large portion sizes have become. Although restaurant portion sizes have increased from one-fourth to three times what they were a decade ago, 62% of the 1,003 people who were interviewed believed restaurant food portions were the same size or smaller during the specified time frame. In addition, 80% of these same people perceived that portion sizes at home were the same size or smaller than they were a decade before. Here are some facts that show how mistaken these people were:

- The average dinner plate is 7 inches larger than it was forty years ago.

- The average calorie level for a burger, fries, and soda was 590 calories in 1957, compared to 1,550 calories today.

- The average cookie twenty years ago was 1 1/2 inches in diameter and 55 calories, compared to the 3 1/2-inch, 375-calorie cookie of today.

- A turkey sandwich of twenty years ago had 320 calories, compared to the 820 calories of today.

- A Caesar salad twenty years ago was 390 calories, compared to 790 calories for today's salad. Is it surprising that restaurants offer half-salads on the menu?

Understanding accurate food portions

To keep an eye on portions, it is very helpful to measure foods into and onto your personal cups, bowls, and plates. A 1/2 cup portion will look differently in an 8 ounce cup compared to a 32 ounce cup. Take a look at some typical portions using your measuring cups and spoons every three months to sharpen your memory regarding portion sizes.

Another good way to keep track of appropriate portions and servings is to compare them to common items. Try these:

One serving of this food:	Looks like:
3 ounces of cooked meat	Deck of playing cards
1 medium apple, orange, peach, or pear	Tennis ball
1 tortilla	Small plate (7-inch diameter)
1 muffin	Large egg
2 tablespoons peanut butter	Golf ball
1 pancake/waffle	4-inch CD
Corn on the cob	Stick of butter
1 ounce cheese	Four dice
1/4 cup fruit, vegetable, cooked cereal, or cooked pasta	Fist of an average woman's hand
Small potato	Computer mouse
1/2 cup ice cream	Racquetball
French fries	10 pencils, or 20 half pencils
Pizza	1/4 of a 7-inch plate
Hamburger patty	Zip disk
Hamburger with bun	Three Zip disks stacked
Burrito or enchilada	Cordless phone

continued

One serving of this food:	Looks like:
Submarine or deli sandwich	Cordless phone
Dressing for a salad	1 strawberry
Cheese sauce for nachos	2 strawberries

Taking Charge of Your Fast Food Choices

It's up to you to make healthy choices when you are eating at a fast food restaurant. There are many ways you can enjoy a fast food meal without going overboard on fat.

Substitute healthy for high fat

- If the menu item has meat, ask for the leanest meat option.
- Ask for a fresh vegetable salsa or vegetables to replace toppings such as sour cream or cheese.
- Substitute one item for another, like a baked potato for French fries.
- Substitute fruit or milk for the French fries or soda on the combination meals.

Keep sauces in their place

- Ask to have sauces, salad dressings, and gravies served on the side so you have control over how much is added.
- Ask for less or no sauce.
- Choose a sauce other than a cream sauce.
- Ask for a lower-fat option (light or nonfat) of the sauce or dressing.
- Choose sauces or dressings that are tomato based rather than butter or cream based.

Preparation

- Ask the waiter to tell you how the menu item is prepared.
- Ask if the menu item can be prepared without being fried. Instead, request it baked, roasted, or steamed.

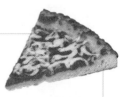

continued

- Eliminate fatty add-ons like cheese, bacon, mayonnaise, and sour cream.
- Ask for your pizza to be baked without grease added to the pan. Choose mushrooms, pineapple, Canadian bacon, or other low-fat toppings.
- Look for code words on a menu that may indicate a lot of fat. See Table 3.1 for the best options.

Table 3.1 Listening for Healthy Fast Food Choices

If You Hear This . . .	Ask Instead for This:
Au gratin	Au jus
Batter dipped	Baked
Breaded	Marinated
Cheesy	Poached
Crispy	Roasted
Rich	Steamed
Stir fried in oil	Broiled
Basted	Herb crusted
Buttery	Fresh
Creamy	Light
Fried	Stir fried
Gravy	Whole grain
Sauteed	Tomato based
Smothered in creme sauce or gravy	Smothered in marinara sauce
Stuffed with cream cheese	Stuffed with feta, cottage cheese, or vegetables

Pay attention to portions

- Order a smaller portion or share it with someone.

- Remember that you can take extra food home with you. Don't feel pressured to eat it all at the restaurant.

- Remove extra chips, rolls, and butter from the table.

Understand what you're ordering

Be familiar with these terms so you can be successful in ordering healthy food (an asterisk indicates the best choices).

Sauces

- Alfredo—a sauce composed of butter, Parmesan cheese, cream, and seasonings

- *Marinara—a sauce composed of tomatoes, onions, garlic, and spices

- Pesto—a sauce made of fresh basil, garlic, oil, pine nuts, and grated cheese

Dressings

- Blue cheese—a cream dressing made with cheese that has been treated with molds to form blue or green veins throughout and give the cheese its characteristic flavor. Some of the more popular of the blues include dana-blu, gorgonzola, Roquefort, and Stilton. Blue cheeses tend to be strong in flavor and aroma, both of which intensify with aging.

- Caesar—garlic vinaigrette dressing (made with Worcestershire sauce and lemon juice) with grated Parmesan cheese.

- *Italian—a salad dressing consisting of olive oil and wine vinegar or lemon juice, seasoned variously with ingredients including garlic, oregano, basil, dill, and fennel.

- Ranch—a creamy salad dressing usually containing milk or buttermilk and mayonnaise.

- *Vinaigrette—a sauce made from oil and vinegar, onions, parsley, and herbs.

Cooking techniques

- *Bake—to cook food in an oven, thereby surrounding it with dry heat.

- *Braise—a cooking method where food (usually meat) is first browned in oil, then cooked slowly in a liquid (wine, stock, or water).

- Bread—to coat food with bread, crackers, or other crumbs, usually by dipping it first into a liquid (beaten eggs, milk, beer, etc.), then into the crumbs, which may be seasoned with various herbs. The breaded food is then fried or baked. Breading helps retain a food's moisture and forms a crisp crust after cooking.

- *Broil—to cook food directly under or above the heat source. Food can be broiled in an oven, directly under the gas or electric heat source, or on a barbecue grill, directly over charcoal or another heat source.

- Fry—to cook food in hot fat over moderate to high heat. Deep-fried food is submerged in hot, liquid fat. Frying (also called *pan frying*) or sautéing refers to cooking food in a lesser amount of fat, which doesn't cover the food. There is little difference in these two terms, though *sautéing* is often thought of as using less fat and being the faster of the two methods.

- *Grill—to prepare food on a grill over hot coals or another heat source. The term *barbecue* is often used synonymously with *grill.*

- *Roast—to oven-cook food in an uncovered pan, a method that usually produces a well-browned exterior and ideally a moist interior. Roasting requires reasonably tender pieces of meat or poultry. Tougher pieces of meat need moist cooking methods such as braising.

- Sauté—to cook food quickly in a small amount of oil in a skillet or sauté pan over direct heat.

Compare and Choose

Now that you know more about food preparations and portions, put your knowledge to work the next time you visit a fast food restaurant. Use Table 3.2 to compare some of the most popular choices at McDonald's, Subway, Wendy's, Quizno's, and Burger King. You can see that simple decisions can make big differences in the calories and fats that you take in. If you prepare beforehand, you can easily make better choices that are tasty and enjoyable.

Table 3.2 Comparing Your Fast Food Options

Restaurant	Food	Calories	Total Fat (g)	Saturated Fat (g)	Carbohydrate (g)	Protein (g)
McDonalds	Hamburger	260	9	3.5	33	13
	Big Mac	560	30	10	47	25
	California Cobb Salad with Grilled Chicken	270	11	5	11	33
	California Cobb Salad with Crispy Chicken	370	18	6	23	29
	Egg McMuffin	290	11	4.5	30	17
	Sausage Biscuit	410	26	8	34	10
	Fruit & Yogurt Parfait (5.3 oz.)	160	2	1	31	4
	McFlurry with OREO (12 oz.)	560	16	9	88	14
Subway	Savory Turkey Breast sandwich	280	4.5	1.5	47	20
	Cheese Steak sandwich	360	10	4.5	47	24
	Chicken and Bacon Ranch sandwich	530	25	10	47	36

EAT RIGHT! HEALTHY EATING IN COLLEGE AND BEYOND

Restaurant	Food	Calories	Total Fat (g)	Saturated Fat (g)	Carbohydrate (g)	Protein (g)
	Grilled Chicken and Baby Spinach salad (no dressing)	140	3	1	11	20
	Tuna with Cheese salad (no dressing)	360	29	6	12	16
Wendy's	Jr. Burger	280	9	3.5	34	15
	Classic Single with Everything	430	20	7	37	25
	Ultimate Chicken Grilled	360	7	1.5	44	31
	Spicy Chicken Fillet	510	19	3.5	57	29
	Frosty (12 oz.)	330	8	5	56	8
	Low Fat Strawberry Yogurt	90	1	0	16	4
Quizno's Sub Sandwich	Small Sierra Smoked Turkey (Raspberry Sauce)	350	6	0	53	23
	Small Honey Bourbon Chicken	359	6	1	45	24
	Small Turkey Lite	334	6	1	52	24

Restaurant	Food	Calories	Total Fat (g)	Saturated Fat (g)	Carbohydrate (g)	Protein (g)
Burger King	Whopper with everything	700	42	13	52	31
	Whopper (no mayonnaise)	540	24	10.5	52	31
	Whopper Jr. with mayo	390	22	7	31	17
	Whopper Jr. (no mayo)	310	13	5.5	31	17
	Original Chicken Sandwich with mayo	560	28	2	52	25
	Original Chicken Sandwich (no mayo)	450	16	0	52	25
	Fire Grilled Chicken salad (no dressing)	190	7	3	9	25
	Tender Crisp (Chicken) Garden Salad (no dressing)	410	22	5	28	25
	Fat Free Honey Mustard Dressing	70	0	0	18	0
	Vanilla Shake (small)	400	15	10	57	8
	Hershey Sundae Pie	300	18	10	31	3

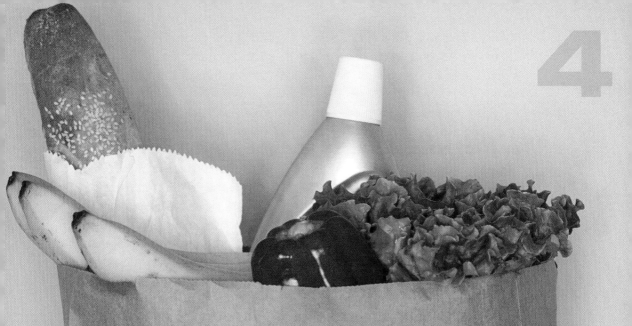

4

Budget Basics
Good Eating for Less

Heidi LeBlanc

Nedra K. Christensen

Meagan Wade

Making a nutritious diet into a top priority will bring you good health and save you money. As you start out on your own, it's more important than ever to invest in your health with good food, and a healthy diet can help while your finances are tight.

Research has found that sensory characteristics (taste, texture, touch, smell, and aesthetics) and cost are the predominant factors that affect a person's food choice. These factors are often barriers to the adoption of a healthy diet because of the misperception that a healthful diet is more expensive and less enjoyable than a diet that doesn't follow nutritional guidelines. Lack of time, lack of money, and lack of nutrition education can act to prevent the consumption of proper foods for optimal health.

Most students find themselves with late nights, busy schedules that include both work and school, and limited time to eat, let alone prepare a nutritious, well-balanced meal. Does this sound familiar? Food consumption often comes down to one word: convenience. The ironic trade-offs for convenience are price and nutrition: you save time, but you compromise your nutrition and you spend more on convenience foods than if you prepared them yourself. It is much more expensive to rely on convenience meals than to add fresh produce and dairy products to your diet. Investing money in health by choosing nutrient-dense products is crucial to optimal functioning and physical and emotional well-being.

Smart Shopping

When money and time are limited, how can I buy healthier foods?

Shopping wisely is the first step to saving money and having a nutritious diet. Two tools to use at the grocery store will help you determine the best value for your money: *unit pricing* to compare similar products, and *price per serving* to compare different foods that serve the same purpose in a meal.

Unit price can be figured by dividing the price of the item by the volume/weight of the contents or number of items in the package. Typically, but not always, buying items in bulk will save more money because the unit price is lower. For example, buying a larger can of beans as opposed to a smaller can will usually have a cheaper per unit price and therefore be a better value. However, be wise about your bulk purchases. Buying too much of a perishable item will most likely result in waste unless it can be frozen, or can be stored for a long period of time.

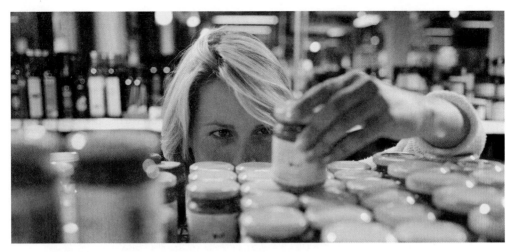

Compare prices and quantities to be a smart shopper.

The unit price can also help when you are trying to decide between two different brands of the same product. The generic brands are typically, but not always, cheaper per unit than name-brand products, though they are often the same quality. For example, when shopping for peanut butter, check the shelf; it usually has cost per ounce. In a recent survey, Skippy was $2.79 for 18 ounces; the unit price is $.15 per ounce. Western Family (a generic brand) was $1.95 for 18 ounces; the unit price is $.11 per ounce. Jif was $2.65 for 18 ounces; the unit price is $.14 per ounce. Adams was $2.79 for 16 ounces; the unit price is $.17 per ounce. As you check the unit price, check the size of container; it was a little confusing that Adams has less in its jar because the jar actually looked bigger than the others. Compare size, cost, taste, and quality.

Price per serving is useful when looking at two different forms of the same product. For example, a bag of potatoes is far different than a box of mashed potato flakes. A 20-pound bag of potatoes will make about fifty servings of potatoes. If that bag costs $2.98, each serving costs about 6 cents. A box of potato flakes makes thirty-four servings and costs $3.89, making each serving cost about 11.4 cents. With a serving of potato flakes costing almost twice as much as a serving of fresh potatoes, the purchase of fresh potatoes would be wiser for a better value.

The price per serving comparison is also useful when comparing two very different products that serve the same function. For example, hamburgers or hot dogs for your next cookout? Four hamburgers made from a pound of beef that costs $1.04 per pound means that the per serving cost is 26 cents. A hot dog from a $1.60 package of eight (for a per serving cost of 20 cents) would be cheaper than a hamburger.

How can I get the most from my food dollar?

Plan ahead

- Create a list of meals and snacks for several days at once.

- Begin planning with the evening meal. This is usually when you will have the most time, so try to pack it with high nutrient dense foods. This is when the family is all together, so the meal is important both socially and nutritionally.

- Plan breakfast next. It is an important meal but is often skipped. It is easier to eat breakfast when you have planned for it.

- Plan lunch and snacks after dinner and breakfast, and fill in with the food groups that are lacking in the other two meals.

- Include all of the food groups: breads, cereals, rice, and pasta; vegetables; fruit; milk, yogurt, and cheese; and meat, poultry, fish, dry beans, eggs and nuts.

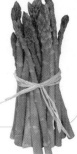

At home, check . . .

- Food you have on hand and what you will need.

- Newspaper ads for weekly specials.

- Coupons for items you use.

38

Decide and write

- Grocery list

- Price next to items on the list that are on sale

Be prepared

- Take your list and coupons with you.

- Avoid shopping when hungry, tired, or rushed.

At the grocery store

- Stick to your list.

- Compare prices (store brands and sale items).

- Check higher and lower shelves for less costly items.

- Shop only aisles with the items you need to get.

At home

- Handle and store food properly to reduce waste.

What are some other ways I can stretch my food dollar?

In addition to comparing prices and making a good shopping list, these strategies will help you get the most for your money:

- Many foods that are already prepared (sandwiches, presliced cheese, bagged salads, etc.) cost much more than those that you prepare yourself. One way to save: instead of buying precut produce, chop a head of lettuce and other vegetables ahead of time so they are ready to use.

- Go for generic and store brands—the product is usually exactly the same as or very similar to name-brand products. The higher price for the brand-name product usually goes toward marketing and advertising, not the quality of the product.

- Keep an ongoing list on the fridge of things that you need to purchase at the store, and commit to stick to that list! Stores are great at marketing their products and strategically placing items in certain places to tempt you to spend more money on "impulse buys." Studies show that shopping without a list can lead consumers to spend twice as much as their shopping trip would have originally cost.

- Visit the store only once or twice a week. Research has demonstrated that more visits to the grocery store mean more unnecessary spending due to impulse buys and lack of planning.

- If you know that you consume a lot of a certain item, stock up when it goes on sale. You can even stock up on perishable items, like meat, if you have a place to freeze them.

- Don't assume that sale items are the best deal. Sometimes these prices are still higher than generic or bulk versions of the same product.

- Plan your menu for an entire week so that you can buy the exact amount needed at a certain time in the week. Some ingredients may be used for more than one meal, which would be ideal!

- Clip coupons only for products you know you will buy and use. Don't let advertisements convince you to buy something you do not really need because it is cheap.

- Explore the local farmers' market. The produce is typically fresher, tastes better, may be cheaper, and directly benefits the farmers by cutting out the middle man.

- Buy fruit in season. An item is "in season" when it is at the peak of its growing season, the most ripe and the most flavorful, and the least expensive.

- Cook from scratch instead of purchasing mixes or premade items, like pancakes or waffles.

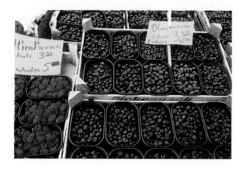

Farmers' markets have fresh and seasonal produce, often at lower prices than supermarkets.

- Make more food than you know you will eat at one meal. Either use the leftovers later that week or freeze them for use later in the month.

- Eat before going to the store; otherwise, food items that are not on the list promise to be more of a temptation, gradually eliminating more and more money from an already thin wallet.

Making a shopping list

Try to follow the guidelines of MyPyramid with menus that provide at least the minimum servings suggested. (The following information is for a 2,000 calorie diet. Go to www.mypyramid.gov to find amounts that are appropriate for you.)

- Grains: eat 6 oz. every day, making at least half of them whole grains.

- Vegetables: eat 2 1/2 cups daily, focusing on getting a variety of color, particularly vegetables that are dark green and/or orange in color.

- Fruits: eat 2 cups daily, going easy on the fruit juices.

- Milk: get 3 cups every day, focusing on lower-fat or fat-free products. If you can't or don't consume milk, choose other products that are high in calcium like fortified cereals and beverages.

- Meat and beans: eat 5 1/2 oz. daily, choosing low-fat or lean meats and poultry. Vary your routine a bit and include things like fish, nuts, beans, peas, and seeds. They make good add-ins or toppings on main dishes.

Keep a list on the fridge with general shopping categories to keep track of what you'll need for the week's menu. These categories could be *produce, meat, dairy, bakery/baking, dry goods, canned goods, frozen,* and *cleaning supplies.* Then, use the shopper's checklist below to make sure you haven't forgotten anything and to give you new ideas for items to try out.

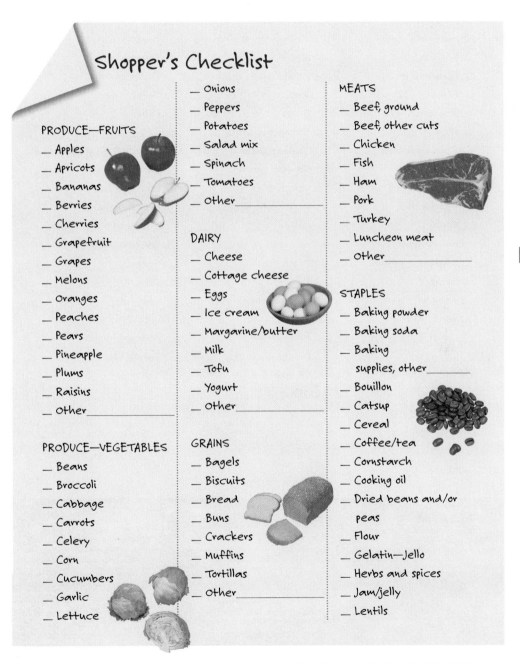

Shopper's Checklist

PRODUCE—FRUITS
__ Apples
__ Apricots
__ Bananas
__ Berries
__ Cherries
__ Grapefruit
__ Grapes
__ Melons
__ Oranges
__ Peaches
__ Pears
__ Pineapple
__ Plums
__ Raisins
__ Other_____

PRODUCE—VEGETABLES
__ Beans
__ Broccoli
__ Cabbage
__ Carrots
__ Celery
__ Corn
__ Cucumbers
__ Garlic
__ Lettuce

__ Onions
__ Peppers
__ Potatoes
__ Salad mix
__ Spinach
__ Tomatoes
__ Other_____

DAIRY
__ Cheese
__ Cottage cheese
__ Eggs
__ Ice cream
__ Margarine/butter
__ Milk
__ Tofu
__ Yogurt
__ Other_____

GRAINS
__ Bagels
__ Biscuits
__ Bread
__ Buns
__ Crackers
__ Muffins
__ Tortillas
__ Other_____

MEATS
__ Beef, ground
__ Beef, other cuts
__ Chicken
__ Fish
__ Ham
__ Pork
__ Turkey
__ Luncheon meat
__ Other_____

STAPLES
__ Baking powder
__ Baking soda
__ Baking
   supplies, other_____
__ Bouillon
__ Catsup
__ Cereal
__ Coffee/tea
__ Cornstarch
__ Cooking oil
__ Dried beans and/or
   peas
__ Flour
__ Gelatin—Jello
__ Herbs and spices
__ Jam/jelly
__ Lentils

41

Shopper's Checklist continued

__ Macaroni
__ Mac/cheese dinners
__ Mayonnaise
__ Mixes, baking
__ Mixes, other
__ Mustard
__ Noodles
__ Peanut butter
__ Pepper
__ Powdered milk
__ Rice
__ Salad dressing
__ Salt
__ Shortening/oil
__ Spaghetti
__ Sugar
__ Brown sugar
__ Powdered sugar
__ Syrup
__ Vinegar
__ Yeast, dry
__ Other_____

CANNED GOODS
__ Applesauce
__ Baked beans

__ Beans (kidney, black, refried)
__ Fruit
__ Fruit juices
__ Main dishes (Spaghetti-O's, ravioli, etc.)
__ Meat (tuna, chicken, etc.)
__ Soups
__ Spaghetti sauce
__ Tomato paste
__ Tomato sauce
__ Vegetables
__ Vegetable juices
__ Other _____

FROZEN FOODS
__ Dinners
__ Fish/seafood
__ Juice
__ Meat items
__ Potato products
__ Vegetables
__ Other_____

PAPER PRODUCTS
__ Bags, paper
__ Bags, garbage
__ Facial tissue
__ Foil
__ Napkins
__ Paper towels
__ Plastic wrap
__ Toilet paper
__ Other_____

HOUSEHOLD STAPLES
__ Bleach
__ Cleanser
__ Dish detergent
__ Dishwasher detergent
__ Laundry detergent
__ Soap
__ Other_____

MISCELLANEOUS
__ Personal hygiene
__ Snack foods
__ Other_____

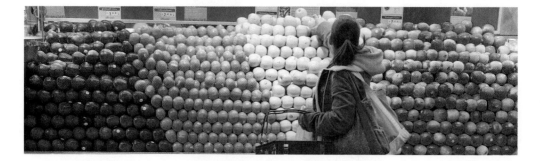

Shop by season

It's important to include fresh fruits and vegetables in your diet. They are more available and cheaper if you buy them in season. See Table 4.1 for a guide to what's fresh when.

Table 4.1 Seasonal Fruits and Vegetables Chart

Fruit	Winter (December– February)	Spring (March– May)	Summer (June– August)	Fall (September– November)
Apple				x
Apricots			x	
Avocado	x	x		
Banana	x	x	x	x
Blackberries, raw		x	x	
Blueberries		x	x	
Cantaloupe			x	
Cherries, sour			x	
Cherries, sweet			x	
Dates, dried			x	x
Elderberries		x	x	
Figs, raw			x	
Gooseberries		x	x	
Grapefruit, pink and red	x			
Grapes			x	x
Honeydew			x	
Kiwi				x

continued

Fruit	Winter	Spring	Summer	Fall
Lemon	x	x	x	x
Lime	x	x	x	x
Mango		x	x	
Nectarine			x	
Orange, navel	x	x	x	
Peach			x	
Pear	x			x
Pineapple	x	x	x	x
Plums			x	
Pomegranate				x
Raspberries		x	x	
Strawberries		x	x	
Tangerine	x			x
Watermelon			x	
Artichoke			x	
Asparagus		x		
Beets		x	x	
Broccoli	x	x		x
Brussels sprouts	x			x
Carrots				x
Cauliflower	x			x
Celery				x
Corn			x	

EAT RIGHT! HEALTHY EATING IN COLLEGE AND BEYOND

Fruit	Winter	Spring	Summer	Fall
Cucumber		X	X	X
Eggplant			X	
Green beans			X	
Leeks			X	X
Lettuce, iceberg		X		X
Lettuce, romaine				X
Mushrooms, raw	X			X
Okra		X	X	X
Peas, green		X		
Peppers, sweet			X	
Potato			X	X
Spinach	X	X		X
Squash, winter				X
Sweet potato	X			X
Tomato			X	
Turnip		X		
Zucchini			X	

Cooking 101

What do I need to start cooking from scratch?

Cooking from scratch is easier if your kitchen is equipped with the proper ingredients and tools. The basic pantry should have the following items:

- Extracts: maple, vanilla

- Oils: olive, sesame, peanut, vegetable, shortening

- Spices: basil, oregano, parsley, thyme, mustard powder, nutmeg, paprika, cinnamon, salt, pepper, garlic powder/salt

- Staples: corn starch, baking powder, baking soda, flour, sugar (powdered, granulated, and brown), yeast, stock (chicken and beef), milk, butter, eggs, mustard, mayonnaise, garlic, onions, lemon juice

The proper cooking tools are also essential to making the most of your time in the kitchen. Though it may seem overwhelming to buy all of these tools immediately, you can gradually acquire them as you go:

- Two saucepans (one small and one large)
- Skillet with a lid
- Glass or metal rectangular and square 2-quart baking dishes
- Baking sheet
- Round cake pans
- Muffin tin
- Pie tin
- Loaf pan
- Can opener
- Set of sharp knives
- Measuring cups and spoons
- Liquid measuring cup
- Ladle
- Spatula
- Whisk
- Slotted spoon
- Wooden spoons
- Grater
- Peeler
- Thermometer
- Colander
- Cutting boards
- Mixing bowls
- Rolling pin
- Pastry blender
- Basket steamer
- Blender

For quick and fun snacks, you will want:

- Air popcorn popper
- Sandwich maker
- Waffle iron

When I cook from scratch, it takes too much time. How can I minimize the amount of time I spend in the kitchen?

One of the most discouraging factors in cooking from scratch is the extra time it takes to prepare the meal. If you follow these tips, the extra time you invest up front will allow you to cook quickly from scratch when time is short. Try to set aside an hour or so after grocery shopping to prepare purchased items for consumption the next week.

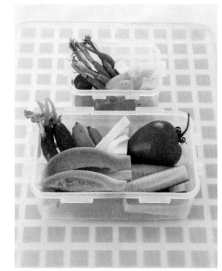

- Cut up vegetables and fruit ahead of time to speed up salad making or inclusion in other dishes. Store in Ziploc bags or Tupperware so they don't dry out.

- Instead of buying cheese singles or pregrated cheese, slice or grate a block of cheese, and wrap it well or freeze it.

Cutting up vegetables ahead of time saves time when you're ready to cook.

- Rather than buying breakfast bars, pour some cereal into small Ziplocs for an easy snack.

- Make a pancake/waffle mix and store it in a large bucket for quick breakfasts.

- For easy breakfasts, premeasure the amount of oatmeal used every morning into individual Ziplocs so it can be grabbed, poured into a bowl, mixed with water, and then put in the microwave for quick cooking.

- Preboil eggs for breakfast or to add to salads or sandwiches.

- "Cook once, eat twice." Plan several meals for the week around a main ingredient that can be cooked and then used in several different ways throughout the week. Ground beef can be cooked and then used in a casserole, in tacos, in soups . . . the possibilities are endless! Cooked pasta can be used for spaghetti, soup, a pasta salad, and so on. Cooking these items in advance will save you lots of time. Be sure you store the items properly so that food safety is not compromised.

- Premake sandwiches for the week, and place them back in the bread bag to keep them fresh. They are easy to grab for any meal or a snack.

When you are just starting out

There are many quick and easy recipes and dishes for people who are just beginning to learn how to cook from scratch.

- Grilled cheese (see recipe) and soup
- Spaghetti or noodles with sauce
- Bagel pizza/tortilla pizza wrap
- Burrito (see recipe)
- Yogurt or cottage cheese with granola, cereal, or fruit
- Quick oats (see recipe)

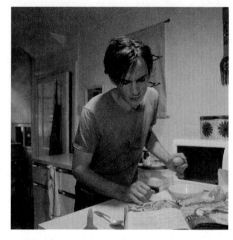

Simple recipes make cooking from scratch easy.

48

Grilled Cheese

2 slices of bread
Pat of butter
1 slice of cheese

Butter the outside of the bread. Place one buttered slice in frying pan, then top with cheese and the other slice of bread. Cook at medium-low heat. Flip over and toast the other slice. Do not overcook.

Burritos

Beans (canned)	Olives
Rice	Salsa
Cheese (grated)	Onions (chopped)
Fresh bell peppers (chopped)	Tortillas
Pimentos	

Mix and match your favorite ingredients from the list above and make a burrito. The same ingredients can be used in a casserole.

Tortilla Casserole

1 cream of mushroom soup (15 oz. can)	Salsa (15 oz.—use cream of mushroom
1 can chicken	can as your measurement tool)
2 cups tortilla chips	Olives (optional) as a garnish
1/4 cup cheese	Green onions (optional) as a garnish

Turn oven on to 400°F. In a casserole dish, mix chicken and cream of mushroom soup, and then top with tortilla chips and cheese. Bake for fifteen minutes or until warm. After cooking, add fresh salsa, olives, and green onions for taste and aesthetics.

Quick Oats

Oatmeal is another way to save money. It's easy to make your own mix so that you can have the convenience of the prepackaged servings.

To prepare a half-dozen bags, first combine 4 cups of old-fashioned rolled oats (not quick-cooking oats) and 3/4 teaspoon of salt in the food processor or blender, and grind them (in two batches, if necessary) to the consistency of wheat germ. Scoop half-cup portions into separate resealable plastic bags. Flavor each one (try the mix-ins below, or make up your own combinations), then seal the bags and shake them to mix.

To prepare, empty the contents of one bag into a bowl and slowly stir in 1 cup of boiling water. Cover and let it sit for three minutes. Stir again and add a splash of milk, if you like, just before serving.

Fast Oatmeal Flavors

Apple cranberry: 1 teaspoon of packed brown sugar and 1 tablespoon each of chopped dried cranberry and apples (can just make apple cinnamon as well)

Brown sugar spice: 1 teaspoon of packed brown sugar and a dash each of ground cinnamon, nutmeg, and clove

Cherry: 1 teaspoon of packed brown sugar and 1 tablespoon dried cherry

Cinnamon raisins: 1 teaspoon of sugar, 1 tablespoon of raisins, and a dash of cinnamon

Pecan delight: 1 teaspoon of packed brown sugar and 1 tablespoon of chopped pecans

Will I really save money cooking from scratch?

It might seem like a lot of effort to make meals from scratch instead of buying prepackaged items. But consider the savings of just one dish made from scratch: a single-serving package of frozen lasagna will cost between $2.50 and $5.00 at the supermarket (23 to 45 cents an ounce for an 11-ounce serving). But you can make lasagna from scratch that will cost $5.50 for the ingredients and make enough servings for you to have leftovers all week.

This recipe is just one example of the savings you'll discover when you start cooking from scratch:

Lasagna

1/2 lb. ground beef	1/2 lb. mozzarella cheese
1 teaspoon garlic powder	12 oz. cottage cheese
1 cup tomato sauce	1/2 cup parmesan cheese
2 1/2 cups canned tomatoes	1 package no-boil lasagna noodles
1/4 teaspoon pepper	

Turn oven on to 350°F. Brown the ground beef. Mix garlic, pepper, tomato sauce, and tomatoes. Mix cheeses. In a 9 x 13 inch pan, layer a thin amount of sauce, noodles, ground beef, and cheese. Repeat to have at least 2–3 layers. Cover with foil and bake thirty-five minutes. Remove foil and cook for ten more minutes. Makes 8–12 servings.

How Do I Put This All Together?

Now that you have learned about menu planning and shopping on a budget, here is a sample one-week menu, a shopping list, and the recipes you need to get started.

Sunday

Breakfast   Pancakes with eggs (freeze leftovers for breakfast on Thursday)
Lunch   Sandwich—peanut butter and jelly
Dinner   Chicken and vegetable stir-fry (one-half bag frozen vegetables)
              Rice (cook extra and refrigerate leftovers for Monday)
              Orange slices

Monday

Breakfast   Cold cereal with orange juice

Lunch   Wrap—lunchmeat, cheese, lettuce, tomatoes, and dressings in a tortilla

Dinner   Zucchini casserole (use 1 cup cooked rice from Sunday)
Corn
Bread with margarine
Milk

Tuesday

Breakfast   Yogurt with banana

Lunch   Sandwich—tuna and lettuce

Dinner   Mexican chicken with beans
Baked potato
Frozen mixed vegetables (half-bag)
Corn muffins
Milk

Wednesday

Breakfast   Oatmeal and orange juice

Lunch   Sandwich—pepperoni, turkey, and ham, with lettuce, tomatoes, cheese, and dressings

Dinner   Spaghetti with meat sauce
Bread with margarine
Salad with dressing
Peas
Milk

Thursday

Breakfast   Leftover pancakes

Lunch   Sandwich—egg salad

Dinner   Chicken divan
Salad with dressing
Baked potato
Milk

Friday

Breakfast   Cold cereal with orange juice

Lunch   Chef salad with all the fixings

Dinner   Enchilada pie
Corn
Bread with margarine
Milk

Saturday

Breakfast   Granola with glass of milk
Lunch   Leftover enchilada pie
Dinner   French toast with syrup
               Fresh fruit (in season)
               Milk

Shopping List

_ Oranges (10–12)
_ Bananas (6–8)
_ Salad mix (2 pounds)
_ Potatoes (5 pounds)
_ Onions (2 medium)
_ Zucchini (1 medium)
_ Tomatoes (1 or 2)
_ Frozen corn (16 oz.)
_ Frozen peas (10 oz.)
_ Frozen mixed vegetables (16 oz.)
_ Stir-fry frozen veggie mix (1 1/2 pounds)
_ Frozen broccoli (10 oz.)
_ Frozen orange juice concentrate (2–12 oz.)
_ Yogurt (32 oz. container)
_ Mayo or Miracle Whip (1 bottle)

_ Milk (3 gallons)
_ Margarine (1 pound)
_ Eggs (18)
_ Cheddar cheese (1 pound or less)
_ Lunchmeats (pepperoni, ham, turkey, roast beef, and the like=1 package)
_ Tuna fish (2 cans)
_ Lean ground beef (3–4 pounds)
_ Chicken, boneless skinless (3 pounds)
_ Spaghetti noodles (12 oz.)
_ Spaghetti sauce (26 oz. jar)
_ Enchilada sauce (10 oz. can)
_ Salsa (20 oz.)
_ Tomato sauce (two 8 oz. cans)
_ Tomato soup (15 oz. can)

_ Cream of chicken soup (15 oz. can)
_ Bread (1–2 loaves)
_ Rice (5 pounds)
_ Pancake mix (56 oz.)
_ Cold cereal in bags (35–40 oz.)
_ Oatmeal (42 oz.)
_ Peanut butter (1 jar)
_ Flour tortillas (1 package)
_ Pinto beans (two 16 oz. cans)
_ Corn muffin mix (2 small boxes)
_ Low-fat salad dressing (16 oz.)
_ Syrup (24 oz.)

Estimated total cost: $60.25 (without tax)

52

Chicken Divan

10 oz. frozen broccoli

1 can cream of chicken soup

1/2 cup shredded cheddar cheese

2 cups diced, cooked chicken

1/3 cup milk

1. Cook broccoli according to package directions. Drain and put in baking dish. Top with chicken.
2. Blend soup and milk. Pour over top of broccoli and chicken. Sprinkle with cheese.
3. Bake at 350°F for ten minutes, or until lightly browned.

Mexican Chicken with Beans

Two 16 oz. cans pinto beans

1 pound boneless, skinless chicken

1 cup salsa

1. Drain beans and put in the bottom of a baking dish. Put the chicken on top, and cover with salsa.
2. Cover and bake at 350°F for 25–30 minutes. If desired, bake uncovered the last ten minutes to thicken the juices.

53

Granola

4 cups rolled oats

1/4 cup brown sugar, maple syrup, or honey

1/4 cup oil (safflower or canola)

1/4 cup water

Optional: 1 teaspoon vanilla, 1 teaspoon cinnamon, 1 cup raisins, dried fruit, 1/2 cup sunflower seeds

In a large bowl, combine oats, sugar, and cinnamon (optional). Combine the oil, water, and vanilla (optional). Mix well with oats.

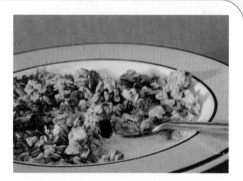

Your own recipe for granola can include your favorite dried fruits and nuts.

Zucchini Hamburger Casserole

1 medium-large zucchini	1 pound ground beef
1 cup chopped onion	1 cup cooked rice
1 teaspoon salt	1/4 teaspoon pepper
8 oz. can tomato sauce	

1. Wash but don't peel zucchini; cut into 3/4-inch cubes.
2. Brown ground beef. Add zucchini and onion. Cook until vegetables are tender.
3. Combine with rest of ingredients, and put in 1 1/2-quart casserole dish.
4. Bake uncovered at 350°F for forty-five minutes.

Yield: Serves 4.

Enchilada Pie

1 pound hamburger	1 large onion
1 package flour tortillas	10 oz. can enchilada sauce
1 can tomato soup	3/4 cup shredded cheddar cheese

1. Chop onion and brown with hamburger. Drain. Stir in enchilada sauce and soup.
2. Cut tortillas into fourths.
3. Layer ingredients: meat, cheese, tortillas, meat, cheese, and tortillas, with a dash of cheese on top.
4. Bake thirty minutes at 350°F.

Yield: Serves 6.

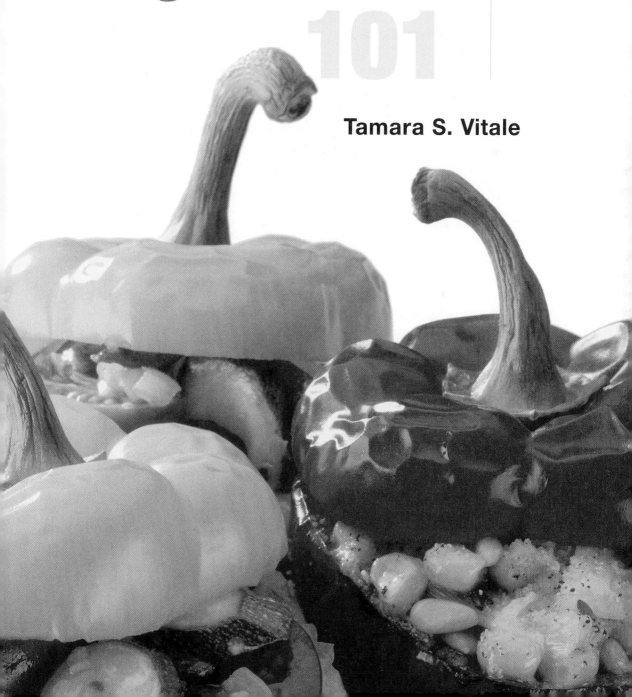

Vegetarianism 101

5

Tamara S. Vitale

Are you a vegetarian or thinking about eating less meat? If so, you are in good company! Famous vegetarians include actress Natalie Portman, musician Moby, and major league baseball manager Tony LaRussa. While these celebrities may have nutritionists, dietitians, cooks, and other experts to help them maintain a healthy meat-free diet, you may need some help making healthy choices. The following questions, answers, and recipes will help you with strategies and guidelines for choosing a vegetarian diet.

Vegetarian Q & A

How many people are vegetarians?

Interest in vegetarian diets continues to grow. Twenty to 25% of adults in the United States report interest in vegetarianism, stating that they eat four or more meatless meals weekly or "usually or sometimes maintain a vegetarian diet" (Ginsberg and Ostrowski 2002). In 2000, approximately 2.5% of the U.S. adult population (4.8 million people) consistently followed a vegetarian diet and affirmed that they never ate meat, fish, or poultry, and about 4% of the Canadian population (about 900,000 people) are vegetarian.

As requests for meatless meals increase, the food industry continues to respond. Most restaurants in the United States now offer vegetarian entrees, fast food restaurants are beginning to offer veggie burgers and other vegetarian options, and most university food services now offer meat-free choices (Vegetarian Resource Group 2000). You'll also find vegetarian products in increasing numbers in most supermarkets. Going meatless for all or some of your meals is becoming more mainstream and is definitely easier than it used to be.

Does vegetarianism have to be "all or nothing"?

No. Dietary choices are personal, whether people choose to eat animal products or not. You may decide to eliminate all animal products, or may omit meat and fish but still include eggs and milk products. You may choose to follow a "plant-based" diet most of the time, but eat an occasional burger at a barbecue or fresh fish while on vacation in Hawaii. Where the lines are drawn regarding dietary "rules" is dependent only on your personal beliefs—it's really no one else's business. There's no reason to attach a label, judge, or convert friends and family, whether it's to a meat-free diet or to a meat-inclusive one. College years are a great time to try on some new behavioral and philosophical hats, as well as some foods and eating styles you've never experienced. But do remember to respect the choices of others; eating is a personal decision but can sometimes seem as controversial as religion and politics!

Will people worry about my health if I'm vegetarian?

Yes, people will worry about you—especially your mom. Vegetarianism is a new concept. Ease her mind by showing her what you're eating instead of meat, not just telling her what you've sworn off. When she realizes that you know what you're doing—and why—she will relax and enjoy that hummus you just learned how to make (see recipe later in this chapter). If you are a guest and your hosts are worried about what to feed you, reassure them that you're flexible and—most importantly—remind them that even if your favorite foods aren't around, nutrient deficiencies don't happen overnight. Whether you eat meat or not is a small factor in the overall spectrum of good nutrition. There are so many other foods out there!

How should a vegetarian eat to avoid nutrient deficiencies?

Not all vegetarian diets are healthy. A meal consisting of a soft drink, fries, and a candy bar is classified as vegetarian, but is loaded with saturated fat and sugar, and short on fiber and many nutrients. But if you added a double cheeseburger on a white bun to that combination, it would still have all of the shortfalls, and be even higher in saturated fat. So the question is not whether eliminating meat is healthier or not; the question is whether you are making wise choices at the fast food order counter. A veggie burger on a whole-grain bun loaded with tomatoes and lettuce, a fruit salad, an order of fries, and bottled water would be healthier and would fit the vegetarian meal bill better.

Substituting piles of grated cheese for meat while avoiding greens and grains is not heading down a healthier highway, either. Follow these tips to make sure that your vegetarian diet is as healthy as possible.

Choose "skinny" milk products
If you like to drink milk and eat yogurt, choose low-fat or nonfat options. That way, you are still getting all of the nutrients like protein and calcium but little or no fat.

Go easy on cheese
It's an easy and readily available protein-rich substitute for meat, but cheese is generally high in saturated fat. A good rule of thumb: add a little grated cheese to your meal only if there is not another source of protein. If you are having a big salad made with lots of veggies, protein add-ons could be garbanzo beans,

sliced hard-boiled eggs, slivered almonds, sunflower seeds, or some cheese, but adding handfuls of all of the above will really add up in calories and fat.

Burritos are often a meal that adds lots of saturated fat to a vegetarian diet. Try adding less cheese and more beans to your bean burritos, which boosts your protein intake without adding a lot of fat.

If you gradually gain weight when you start trying vegetarian meals, these high-fat foods might be something to keep an eye on. You might also want to try some of the reduced-fat cheeses and cottage cheese on the market—they are still great sources of protein but have substantially less fat.

Speaking of beans—eat plenty

Beans are protein powerhouses, have many other vitamins and minerals, and are inexpensive, easy-to-fix additions to vegetarian meals. Canned beans are a great staple to have on hand—just make sure you drain and rinse well before using. This reduces the sodium content as well as the "gas-forming" properties that socially conscious college students would prefer to avoid. Cooking dried legumes (such as pintos, white beans, and black beans) from scratch is simple and even less expensive. (See recipes later in this chapter for details.)

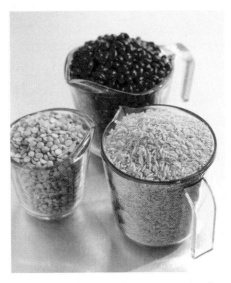

Beans and rice are important parts of a balanced vegetarian diet.

Try adding kidney beans to salads, black beans to nachos or quesadillas, and white beans to spaghetti sauce. You can dip vegetable sticks and pita bread into hummus, which is made from garbanzo beans. There's not a simpler vegetarian entrée than a whole-wheat tortilla topped with refried pinto beans and a sprinkle of cheese, rolled up, microwaved, and enjoyed with plenty of salsa.

Go nuts

Peanut butter, nuts, and seeds are another low-cost, easy way to add protein and many other nutrients to meatless meals. Although they contain fats that are heart healthy, large handfuls eaten often can add more calories to your diet than you might realize. Mix nuts and seeds into a "gorp" mix with whole-grain cereal squares, dried fruit, and a few chocolate chips for a snack that is portable, nutritious, and tasty. If you pre-portion this mix into sealable bags, you can throw it into your backpack or pocket for healthy munchies during the day.

EAT RIGHT! HEALTHY EATING IN COLLEGE AND BEYOND

Incorporate eggs

You may have heard that eggs are high in fat and cholesterol content. But, since you are already limiting saturated fat and cholesterol in your diet by not eating meat, there's definitely room for eggs in a healthy vegetarian diet. They are a rich source of protein, iron, and many other nutrients. Omelets, frittatas, and scrambled egg burritos are quick, easy, and cheap meals. The next time you stir-fry some veggies, scramble a few eggs with a little soy sauce, cut it into cubes, and throw it on top of your bowl of stir-fried vegetables and brown rice. You'll be pleasantly surprised by how easy and delicious your meal is.

If you do wish to limit cholesterol and fat, substitute two egg whites for one whole egg in your cooking and baking. Egg whites do not contain any fat, but are rich in protein.

Do I need to take supplements if I eat a vegetarian diet?

Supplements aren't necessary for vegetarians unless you tend to eat the same limited choices day after day or if you have eliminated major food groups. Consider the overall quality of your diet, and adjust accordingly.

For example, if you eliminate meat but eat plenty of iron-rich foods such as fortified cereals and dark, leafy greens, you shouldn't need a supplement. (Note: supplemental iron should not be taken without a diagnosis of iron-deficiency anemia, whether you are a vegetarian or not.) If you follow a vegan diet but include soy products and fortified cereals, then you don't need a B_{12} supplement.

If you are eating a wide array of fruits and vegetables (that is, if most of your meals are as colorful as a box of Crayolas), this is great insurance that you are getting a wide variety of nutrients. If your plate isn't very colorful, think about which colors are missing and how you can add them. If you don't like carrots, try apricots, mangoes, or sweet potatoes. If colorful foods rarely touch your lips, a multivitamin supplement may be a good idea. This is true for meat eaters as well.

How can I add more plant-based foods into my diet?

As people try to incorporate more plant-based foods into their diets, they sometimes get overwhelmed or think they have to follow a rigid set of rules. Not so! Here are some suggestions to make this transition simpler.

Meatless Monday is a national health campaign to help Americans prevent heart disease, stroke, diabetes, and cancer, four of the leading causes of death in the United States, by cutting down on their unhealthy fat intake. For more information, tips, and recipes, go to www.meatlessmonday.com.

More meatless options are being offered in restaurants—even fast food chains. Ask your waiter (or the chef) for recommendations. Many chains provide ingredient information on their Web sites as well.

Most ethnic restaurants offer vegetarian specialties. Here are some traditional offerings that you may want to try.

- Chinese: egg foo yung, tofu-broccoli stir fry
- French: ratatouille or spinach quiche
- Greek: spanakopita, feta-tomato salad
- Indian: curried eggplant and potatoes, dal with naan
- Italian: pasta primavera, eggplant parmesan
- Mexican: black bean tostada, chiles rellenos
- Middle East: falafel, hummus, tabouli

Adding beans and nuts to a salad helps make it into a complete meal.

Most campus dining halls are offering more vegetarian foods. If yours does not, give some simple suggestions for adding some. Sometimes a few minor adjustments provide major flexibility. Adding some cottage cheese, baked beans, and sunflower seeds to the baked potato bar, and offering tofu as an option at the stir-fry stand, are easy and doable. Food service managers are generally pleased because these additions are very affordable, too—often meat is the most expensive ingredient in a meal. For more suggestions on becoming involved in decisions about campus food offerings, see chapter 1, "Eating Healthy in the Dining Hall."

If you like to cook, check out the frozen foods aisle in your grocery store. Cheese-filled frozen ravioli are quick to fix and delicious enough for company topped with a tomato sauce. Also, you'll be surprised by how much meatless "bacon" and "sausages" the larger supermarkets carry. Most are soy based and are excellent sources of protein.

You can also find meatless "burgers" in your supermarket—two popular brands are Gardenburgers and Boca Burgers. Try a few different brands on a toasted whole-grain bun with plenty of your favorite trimmings, and see which you prefer. See the "Important Ingredients" section later in this chapter for more information on other soy-based products.

Invest in a vegetarian cookbook to expand your food horizons. An excellent reference book for meatless cooking is *Vegetarian Cooking for Everyone* by Deborah Madison (Broadway Books, 1997). Another great cookbook for new and in-a-hurry vegetarians is *The 15-Minute Gourmet: Vegetarian* by Paulette Mitchell (Wiley, 2000).

Making Vegetarian Snacks and Meals

Easy snacks

All of these snacks contain a mix of carbohydrates and protein. Snacks with protein tend to keep you full longer than snacks with carbohydrates alone, and help to ensure that you are getting adequate amounts of protein in a vegetarian diet. Whole-grain carbohydrates also tend to digest more slowly than "white" choices—another way to make that snack last through your exam and keep your brain cells functioning at their best.

- Cut-up fresh fruit topped with vanilla yogurt and cinnamon
- Bagel and low-fat cream cheese
- Trail mix (nuts, seeds, dried fruit, and whole-grain cereal squares)
- Yogurt and granola
- Popcorn sprinkled with parmesan cheese
- Soft pretzels with mustard and cheese slices
- Fruit smoothies (see recipes)
- String cheese and whole-grain crackers
- Graham crackers or bananas spread with peanut butter
- Cottage cheese and canned peaches

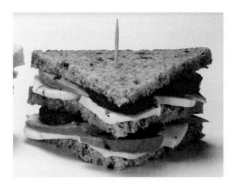

Quick meals

Easy-to-make dinners don't have to be gourmet to be healthy. Grilled cheese sandwiches and canned soups with a green salad and an apple can be a healthy dinner,

Tomatoes, peppers, cheese, and whole-wheat bread add up to a quick snack or meal.

as can microwaved bean burritos, baby carrots, and canned pineapple. If you want to get more advanced, learning how to prepare staples such as rice, pasta, grains, omelets, and roasted vegetables is a huge step toward a nutritious diet and will save you time and money in the long run. A large pasta salad made with lots of vegetables and beans makes great lunches and leftovers. When you rush to the fridge in starving mode after classes, you'll be happy to see it, and you'll save money and be less tempted by the cookie jar, too.

Meal planning is an important part of eating well, and it really doesn't have to be complicated—"meals in minutes" is the name of the game. Try this approach to quick meal planning: choose a carbohydrate (pasta, baked potatoes, bread, etc.), find a vegetable and a fruit, and decide on a simple protein source (milk products, beans, nuts, a soy-based product, etc.). Couldn't be simpler. If in doubt that you are eating enough protein at that meal, drink a glass of milk or soy milk, or have a yogurt for a snack later on.

Here are some ideas for quick meals. Just add the element that is missing— usually a fruit and/or a vegetable.

- Grilled cheese sandwich: add sliced tomatoes when done cooking.
- Mexican egg burrito: scrambled egg with chopped peppers and salsa in a whole-wheat tortilla.
- Pita bread stuffed with hummus, cucumbers, and tomatoes drizzled with any creamy dill dressing.
- Peanut butter and banana sandwich.
- Baked potato with cottage cheese and salsa.
- Quesadillas with black beans, cheese, and tomato slices.
- Peanut butter sandwich on whole-grain bread.
- Bean or minestrone soup with whole-grain crackers.
- Pasta with marinara sauce and white beans.
- Taco salad: greens, black beans, tomatoes, grated cheese, and corn, topped with crumbled chips and salsa.

Important ingredients: Soy and beans

Soy foods and beans are important protein boosters for many vegetarian meals. If you are new to vegetarian cooking, you may not know much about these foods and how to prepare them. Here are some tips.

Choosing soy foods

Soybeans are a widely available and reliable nonmeat protein source, and come in many forms.

- Soy milk: soybeans are ground with water, cooked, and then strained. Many brands are fortified with vitamins and minerals, and soy milk is available in shelf-stable packages as well as in the refrigerated section. Soy milk is also converted into yogurt, sour cream, ice cream, and cheese.

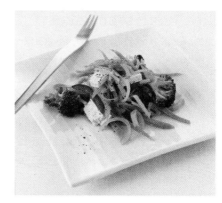

- Tofu: coagulants and heat are added to soy milk to make tofu, which is available in many forms, including silken, extra firm, baked, and marinated. The softer varieties work best in recipes where they are pureed, and the firmer versions are preferred in stir-fries.

Tofu and other soy foods are a great source of protein.

- Tempeh: A fermented soy food with a dense, meaty quality, which can be used to simulate strips of bacon and meats.

- Miso: A flavor paste made from fermented soybeans; it forms the base of many soups as well as soy sauce.

Cooking Dried Beans From Scratch

This hot-soak method is recommended to limit the gas-producing tendencies of beans.

Heat 10 cups water to boiling in a large pot. Add 1 pound (about 2 cups) rinsed and sorted beans (pick out any small sticks or pebbles) and boil 2–3 minutes. Remove from heat, cover, and let soak 4–16 hours. After soaking, drain and rinse the beans, and discard the soaking water. Cover with fresh, cold water (to cover plus 1–2 inches). Add seasonings (see note, below) if you like, and simmer until beans are tender (they should be tender enough to smash against the roof of your mouth with your tongue, but not mushy).

You can also use a pressure cooker to reduce cooking time, or a slow-cooker to allow them to cook while you are gone. Follow the manufacturer's instructions.

When the beans are tender, use immediately in a recipe, refrigerate for a few days, or pack into 2-cup freezer containers or bags and freeze them for future use.

Note: add acidic foods (tomatoes, vinegar, molasses, or salsa) and salt at the end of cooking. If added at the beginning, cooking time will be much longer.

Mexi-bean Bake

6 oz. tortilla chips, broken (or 6–8 corn tortillas, torn)
One 15 oz. can corn (or about 1 1/2 cups frozen corn)
3 cups leftover or canned chili
Shredded cheese (1 to 1 1/2 cups)

Spray an 8 1/2" x 11" baking dish with nonstick cooking spray. Cover bottom of pan with 1/3 chips, then 1/3 corn, 1/3 chili, and 1/3 cheese. Repeat layers two more times. Bake at 350°F for 25–30 minutes. Serve with salsa and sour cream, if desired.

Black Bean Salsa

Serve as a topping for baked potatoes, for quesadillas, mixed with cooked cold pasta for a quick pasta salad, or as a dip.

1 can black beans, drained and rinsed, or 1 1/2 cups cooked dry black beans
One 15 oz. can corn, drained
One 15 oz. can tomatoes with green chilies (or 2–3 fresh tomatoes, chopped)
2 cloves garlic, minced
1/2 bunch cilantro, chopped
1/3 cup onion or green onion, chopped
1 avocado, chopped
Juice of 1 lime
Juice of 1/2 lemon
Dash hot sauce
Salt and pepper to taste

Mix in a large bowl. Cover, and refrigerate for 2–3 hours to blend the flavors (if you can resist).

Hummus

Purchased hummus is great—but if you have a little time and want to save money, fresh hummus is even more delicious and is a great snack to make for a party.
Yield: about 3 cups

Two 16 oz. cans garbanzo beans, drained and rinsed
3 cloves garlic, peeled
1/3 cup tahini (sesame seed paste)
1 tsp. salt
Juice of 1 lemon
1/4 tsp. cayenne pepper, ground
1/4 tsp. cumin, ground

continued

1/4 tsp. black pepper, ground

1/3 cup extra virgin olive oil

1 handful parsley

3-4 green onions, cut into 1" pieces

Water as needed (approx 1/3 cup)

Place all ingredients in a food processor or blender. Add water as needed to form a smooth paste. Adjust seasonings to taste.

Garnish with parsley if desired. Serve with pita bread wedges and fresh vegetables.

Tropical Surprise Smoothie

Makes 1 serving—approximately 1 1/2 cups

1 cup vanilla fat-free yogurt

1/2 cup crushed pineapple (not drained)

1 kiwi, peeled

1 frozen banana

Place all ingredients in a blender. Blend until smooth. Serve immediately.

Tip: don't EVER throw away an overripe banana! Simply peel and freeze in a Ziploc baggie. You'll be glad you have a stash when you get a craving for one of these yummy smoothies.

Berry Blast Smoothie

Makes 1 serving—approximately 1 1/2 cups

1 cup strawberry fat-free yogurt

1 cup fresh or frozen mixed berries (strawberries, boysenberries, raspberries, etc.)

2 tbsp. frozen orange juice concentrate

3 drops almond extract

Place all ingredients in a blender. Blend until smooth. Serve immediately.

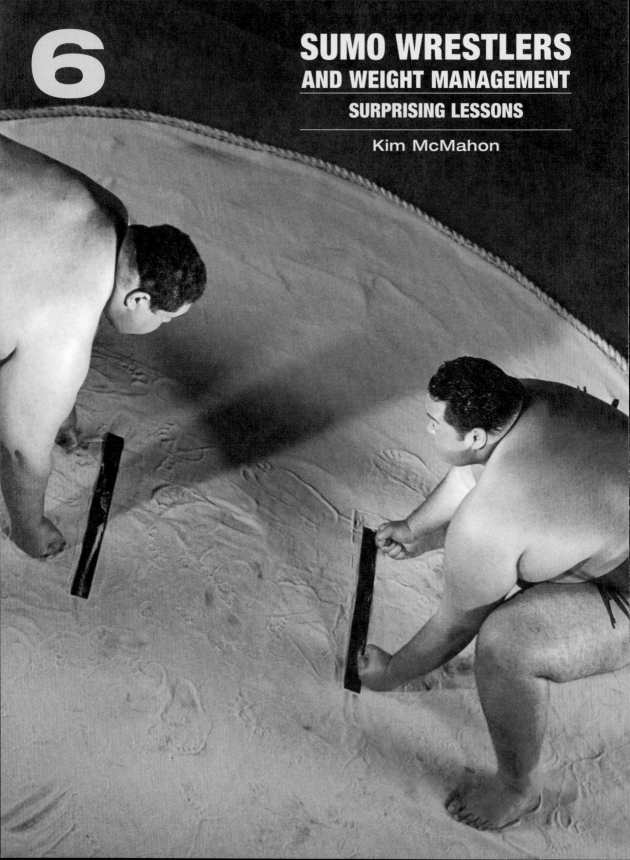

6

SUMO WRESTLERS
AND WEIGHT MANAGEMENT
SURPRISING LESSONS

Kim McMahon

Is it possible to work out 3–5 hours a day, seven days a week, eat a relatively low-fat diet, and still gain weight? Yes—sumo wrestlers follow just this plan to pack on the pounds. In their sport, the rules are simple: one of two wrestlers loses when he is forced out of the fifteen-foot wrestling ring or if anything other than his feet touch the playing surface. The heavier the fighter, the lower his center of gravity, and therefore the tougher it is to force him out of the ring, so wrestlers want to be as big as possible. The average sumo wrestler stands about 6 feet tall and weighs 336 pounds, with the largest wrestler in sumo history tipping the scales at 680 pounds. Naturally, sumo wrestlers have large body frames and some genetic tendencies to help them become as massive as a large sea animal, but it also takes a great deal of dedication to a particular lifestyle in order to pack on the pounds. A sumo wrestler's diet is a huge part of the reason why they can gain so much weight. For those of us who want to lose weight or simply not gain, there are lessons to be learned from some of the world's "biggest" weight experts. Whatever these men are doing, we should be doing just the opposite.

The Importance of What and When You Eat

Does the timing of your meals affect your weight?

Sumo wrestlers sure think so. They claim it is not just what they eat that makes them gain weight, but also how and when they eat. Wrestlers live and train together, sharing duties of cleaning and preparing meals, with one big meal and one smaller meal per day.

The menu has little variation: *chanko-nade,* a single-pot stew made mainly of pork, cabbage, eggs, and bean sprouts, is served every day as the main mid-morning meal. This meal is eaten after the morning workout, followed by a nap, some leisure time, a less elaborate dinner, and free time. When curfew arrives, the married wrestlers go home to their families and the single men return to their rooms. The wrestlers do not eat again until after a good night's sleep, morning duties, morning workout, and then the next *chanko-nade* feast.

The *chanko* stew is high in complex carbohydrates, protein, and vegetables, making it similar to the diet followed by other, smaller Japanese people. So if these wrestlers are eating the same types of foods as smaller people who share their same customs, how is it possible for them to gain so much weight? The answer has to do with *when* and *how much* they are eating.

Think of the mass of a sumo wrestler. If an average man needs about 1 calorie per kg of body weight per hour (.9 kcal per kg of body weight per hour for women) just to maintain his basal metabolic rate (BMR), or resting, functions, how many calories a day does a 336-pound (153 kg) man need? The answer:

1. BMR = (153 kg x 1) x 24 = 3,672 calories.

2. Add the activity level for sumo wrestling as *moderately active* (50%):

   3,672 calories (BMR) x .50 (or 50%) = 1,836 kcal/day

3. Calculate the total daily energy output by adding together BMR and the energy needed to perform daily activities.

   3,672 kcal + 1,836 kcal = 5,508 kcal/day

4. If this person wants to gain weight, add an additional 500 kcal/day.

   5,508 kcal + 500 kcal = 6,008 kcal/day are needed to gain about 1 pound per week.

The wrestlers are getting well over half of their caloric needs from the *chanko* meal all in one sitting. What happens after that? They go for a long period of time without eating, have a significantly smaller evening meal, and then "starve" themselves until the next meal. *Gorgers* are how we describe the way a sumo wrestler eats—going for a long period of time (more than four to five hours) without eating, and then eating past the point of being full. Sound familiar? How often do you skip breakfast, eat a light lunch, and then overeat at dinner? Just the opposite, a person who consistently eats small meals throughout the day is referred to as a *grazer.* Given the same amount of calories, gorgers who eat one or two meals per day will gain 25% more weight than grazers fed the same amount of food in six small meals. If you habitually skip meals, your fat cells become greedy and you start to conserve more calories to protect you from starving to death.

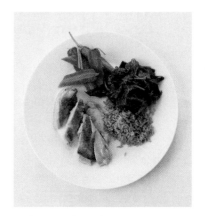

Balanced meals help you get the nutrients you need and avoid overeating.

Our bodies are great at adapting to certain situations; the threat of starvation decreases your metabolism so that you can survive on less calories. If you and a 500-pound sumo wrestler were both stranded on an island without any food, who would live the longest? The sumo wrestler would. First, your bodies would adapt to the sudden decrease in energy intake by slowing down your metabolism so that you are burning less calories to stay alive. Next, after using your carbohydrate energy reserves, your body would use fat stores and start to break down its own protein sources such as muscle and tissue to provide energy that will keep your heart and lungs working. The sumo wrestler would have many more fat stores to live off of on that island.

However, since you are not on an island and since you live in a society where food is plentiful and healthy choices are easy to find, why make your body think starvation is just around the corner? Keep your body well fed by not skipping meals. Do this by including healthy snacks throughout the day. The sumo wrestlers will be doing just the opposite.

How can you determine when you have eaten enough and avoid overeating?

Listen to your body signals that tell you when you are hungry and when you are comfortably full. Honor these feelings. Easier said than done? Next time you sit down to eat dinner, try this: dish up your usual serving size. Eat half of it, stop eating, and turn your attention to something else for about 10–15 minutes. Now, reevaluate your hunger. Are you still hungry? If so, eat half of what you have left and continue this same exercise. If you eat your whole plate and you are still hungry, go ahead and get another serving. If you notice that you are full before you expected, simply cover your remaining food and store it properly. You will likely be hungry again later (OK, probably sooner than later), so you can finish your meal when you get hungry again.

When the eating occasion is finally finished, you may look back and determine that you ate the same amount of food as you would have if you had eaten the meal all at once. One very important component is different—your meal patterning. By grazing instead of gorging, you have spread out the calories and fed your metabolism and your fat cells at a more constant rate without overdoing it. Your metabolism is always running, and you always need some calories to burn. By spreading out the amount of food you eat, you are keeping your fat cells happy and they will not feel the threat of starvation. In addition, keeping your body fed will help you avoid getting too hungry.

What happens when you let yourself get too hungry?

Think of the last time you were really hungry. What did you eat? Something low in fat and high in fiber? Probably not. Most likely, your choice was high in sugar and fat (a brownie, a piece of pizza?). What sounds good when you are "starving" is most likely something that will give you a quick burst of energy (in other words, something high in simple sugars). Once you reach the moment of excessive hunger, your efforts at making moderate and healthy choices easily disappear.

It takes about twenty minutes for your stomach to get the message to your brain that you are full. When you eat quickly without evaluating your fullness, or when you eat until you actually feel full, you have definitely overeaten. How many calories can you overeat in 10–15 minutes? A lot—especially if you end the meal with a high-calorie dessert! Also, when you let yourself get too hungry, you are more likely to eat faster than you are able to evaluate your fullness, leading to overeating. Sumo wrestlers are masters at this. Since they eat only 1–2 times each day, you can guarantee they are pretty hungry when meal time comes around. In an effort to avoid getting too hungry, try not to go longer than four or five hours without eating. This is easily done by including snacks throughout the day.

If I eat with a group of people, will I eat more than when eating alone?

Sumo wrestlers eat together in a social environment. Research shows that eating meals with others can easily result in eating larger quantities and more calories from fat than when eating alone. Eating with friends and family can be a wonderful experience. Simply be aware of your habits when eating with others, and don't lose track of those hunger and fullness signals.

When I think a chocolate candy bar sounds good, should I eat it?

Another important part of listening to your hunger/fullness cues is eating the types of foods you are feeling hungry for. When you feel the first signs of hunger, stop and ask yourself: what really sounds good? Are you in the mood for salty or sweet? Crunchy or soft? Spicy or bland? Eat what you are hungry for and remember to stop eating when you are satisfied, giving yourself permission to eat the rest later.

Can you remember a time when you thought a candy bar sounded good but you ate something "more healthy" instead? Chances are you weren't satisfied and you ate your way straight to the candy bar. First an apple, then some pudding, next a small piece of pumpkin pie, and finally the candy bar. Wouldn't it have been more satisfying to have had the candy in the first place (and look at how many calories you would have saved in the process)?

Why don't I feel satisfied after I finish a meal?

Satiety, or the feeling of fullness you get as you eat, is a very important factor in preventing overeating. Research shows that if you cut calories by eating less food, you will feel hungry and deprived. Eating what you are hungry for will add to your satiety, but there is more to it than food choices.

Suppose you are hungry for a candy bar. You eat a snack-size candy bar and you are still hungry. What next? Not only do we need to satisfy our needs with the *flavor* of foods we feel hungry for, but we also satisfy our needs by eating a particular *amount* of food. Research shows that a person will generally feel full from a particular amount of food. If you choose foods that give you the highest amount of nutrients for the least amount of calories, you are eating a high nutrient-dense food. Take the candy bar, for example. A candy bar has around 270 calories. You could eat the same amount of calories by eating six slices of bacon, four peaches, or twenty

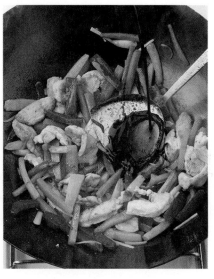

This chicken and vegetable stir-fry has high nutrient density.

cups of leafy green lettuce. If you choose to eat the candy bar, you will probably be hungrier sooner than if you had eaten twenty cups of lettuce. In other words, by choosing foods low in nutrient density, you will need to eat a larger amount to feel satisfied. That larger amount will also add up as more overall calories.

What types of food are high nutrient-dense foods? Fruits, vegetables, whole grains, and low-fat proteins. By incorporating these foods, you increase the nutrient density and lower the calories all at the same time as you increase the amount of food you are eating. Remember the diet of sumo wrestlers; not loaded with fruits and vegetables, is it? Try adding 2–3 more servings of fruits and vegetables to each of your meals in an effort to keep the amount of the food you are eating to a satisfying level while decreasing the overall calories from fat and increasing the vitamin, mineral, carbohydrate, and fiber content of your meals

What are some calorie-conscious food choices?

Try these ideas for healthy snacks

- Make a fruit smoothie by mixing fruit with low-fat yogurt.
- Combine fruit with low-fat cottage cheese or yogurt.
- Make frozen fruit chips by pureeing fruit and then freezing it.
- Spread peanut butter on celery slices.
- Mix low-fat ricotta cheese with unsweetened pineapple and spread on celery.
- Make vegetable kebabs with bell pepper strips, mushrooms, cherry tomatoes, and zucchini chunks. Dip in fat-free salad dressing.
- Dip cinnamon graham crackers in yogurt.
- Munch on string cheese and whole-grain crackers.
- Dip low-fat cookies in 1% or skim milk.
- Spread pizza sauce, toppings, and a thin layer of cheese on a bagel.

Pay attention to your beverages

See Table 6.1 for the details on your favorite drinks and remember these tips:
- Drink water for thirst; add a slice of lemon or lime to perk up the taste.
- Choose low-calorie juices or diet soda instead of high-calorie drinks. Most fruit juice can be diluted with equal parts water for a lower-calorie drink.
- If you drink whole or 2% milk, switch to 1% or skim.

Small changes can add up to big calorie savings

- When baking a cake, brownies, muffins, or quick breads, use applesauce instead of oil.
- Trim visible fat from meat before cooking. After cooking, drain or rinse off fat drippings.
- Have fresh fruit for dessert.

continued

- Go easy on the salad dressing. Try fat-free varieties or oil and vinegar varieties. See Table 6.2 for a comparison of various dressings and condiments.
- Salsa is not just for chips. Use it as a low-calorie and zesty topping on potatoes, vegetables, fish, chicken, eggs, and meat.

Table 6.1 How Many Calories Are in That Glass?

Beverage	Calories per 8 Oz. Serving
Regular soda (cola)	303 (24 oz. serving)*
Whole milk	149
2% milk	122
Fruit juice	120–150
1% milk	102
Skim milk	86
1/2 fruit juice + 1/2 water	60–75
Diet soda (cola)	0
Water with lemon or lime	0

* Many soft drinks are now sold in 24 oz. or larger containers.

Table 6.2 What's Topping Off Your Meal?

Condiment	Calories per 2 Tbsp. Serving
Ranch salad dressing	148
Oil and vinegar dressing	50–60
Reduced-fat salad dressing	35–70
Catsup	32
Fat-free salad dressing	20–45
Salsa	10

Exercise: The Other Half of the Weight Management Equation

Being strong is an important characteristic of any winning sumo wrestler. After all, in order to push over something the size of a refrigerator, you have to be as powerful as one. The exercise they do every day consists of using short bursts of energy similar to what we would describe as lifting weights. Going for a three-mile run or riding a bicycle for sixty minutes is not a priority. In addition, sumo wrestlers spend a lot of time at practice watching other wrestlers and waiting for their turn in the ring. The calories they burn during their exercise sessions do little to offset the amount of calories they eat.

What type of exercise is best for me?

Keep your workouts slow and steady. The most effective type of exercise is any continuous activity where your intensity is about 60–85% of the maximum intensity you can do. You should be able to breathe at a pace that is somewhat labored but still comfortable.

The next time you are exercising, try this talking test to measure your intensity: you should be able to speak three syllables of a sentence before having to take the next breath. For example:

"Old McDonald" [breath] "had a farm" [breath] "E-I" [breath] "E-I" [breath] "OOO."

Adjust the speed of your workout according to how easy or difficult the talk test is.

It is important to keep your body at this pace because aerobic-type exercise not only increases metabolism during a workout, but it also causes your metabolism to stay increased for a period of time after exercising, calling on stored calories for extra fuel and allowing you to burn more calories all of the time.

Examples of aerobic exercise are rapid walking, bicycling, jogging, working on an elliptical machine, swimming, and aerobics class.

Do "lose-weight-quick" products work?

It is easy for some people to lose weight quickly by going on a diet or simply decreasing the amount of food that they eat. Imagine that you are a healthy twenty-year-old woman who is 5'3" and weighs 115 pounds. You have a normal percent body fat at 25%, with 86 pounds of lean body mass. If you consistently eat 100 more calories per day than you burn, at the end of two years you will have gained about twenty pounds, and have a percent body fat of 46% and 89 pounds of lean body mass.

Now, you realize that spring break is only eight weeks away and you want to lose twenty pounds before you and your friends go on a trip. You go on a popular rapid-weight-loss diet. After eight weeks on the diet, you see results (because your caloric intake has been far less than your caloric output) and your weight is back down to 115 pounds. There is a catch: of the twenty pounds you lost, ten pounds were fat, five pounds were water, and five pounds were muscle. Although you are back to your original weight, your percent body fat is now 35% and you have ten pounds less of lean muscle mass. Were you wondering why your "old" jeans don't fit the same? A higher percent body fat equals a larger waist line.

After a very fun spring break trip, you settle back into your more usual diet and slowly begin to gain weight again. If you continue this cycle of dieting and weight changes, your body responds by decreasing the amount of calories you need and therefore decreasing your overall metabolism. Weight loss with exercise can prevent your metabolism from slowing down and will stimulate fat loss, increasing lean muscle mass.

How much exercise do I need to manage my weight?

A difference of about 3,500 calories is needed to change your weight. A medium-sized adult would have to walk more than thirty miles to burn up 3,500 calories, the equivalent of one pound of fat. Although that may seem like a lot, you don't have to walk the thirty miles all at once. Walking a mile a day for thirty days will achieve the same result. Remember, however, not to increase your food intake and negate the effects of walking. Table 6.3 shows the calories you can burn in an hour of some popular activities.

Table 6.3 How Many Calories Am I Burning?

Activity	Calories Burned per Hour
Bicycling 6 mph	240
Bicycling 12 mph	410
Jogging 5.5 mph	740
Jogging 7 mph	920

continued

Activity	Calories Burned per Hour
Jumping rope	750
Running in place	650
Running 10 mph	1,280
Skiing (cross-country)	700
Swimming 25 yds/min	275
Swimming 50 yds/min	500
Tennis (singles)	400
Walking 2 mph	240
Walking 4 mph	440

How do I include activity in my daily life?

Many students find it difficult to fit an exercise program into schedules that already include school, socializing, working, and other activities. A good way to increase your caloric output is by changing your lifestyle to incorporate more activity every day. Don't forget that muscles used in any activity, any time of day, contribute to fitness. Try working in a little more movement with these extras:

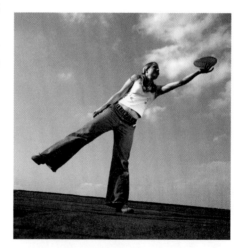

- Take the stairs instead of the elevator.

- Park at the far end of a parking lot and walk to class or to the store.

- Get off the bus a few blocks before your stop.

- When taking study breaks, walk around the library or the block around your apartment.

You can include exercise in your life without participating in an organized sport or joining a gym.

- Increase your pace when cleaning your apartment. Clean areas of your apartment that you usually do not get to.

- Go for a short walk or do some stretching exercises before breakfast and after dinner.
- Change the route you usually take to campus or between classes, adding a walk up a hill when possible.

What precautions should I take when I'm exercising outside?

When it's hot or humid

- Exercise during cooler and/or less humid times of day. Try early morning or evening.
- Drink plenty of fluids, especially water.
- Wear light, loose-fitting clothing.
- Stop exercising at the first sign of muscle cramping or dizziness.
- Find an area where there is a lot of shade, such as a walking path or mountain trail. Again, be sure to bring along and drink plenty of water.

When it's cold

- Dress in layers. You can remove each layer as you need to after you get started.
- Wear gloves or mittens to protect your hands.
- Wear a hat or cap. Up to 40% of body heat is lost through your neck and head.
- Adjust the size of your shoes if you need to wear thicker socks.
- Start your exercise session with a ten minute "warm up."
- Drink plenty of fluids. You can get dehydrated in the winter, too.
- Stop if you experience shivering, drowsiness, or disorientation. You may need help for hypothermia.

How can I exercise on campus or at home?

There are many opportunities for exercise on campus on your own or through your school's physical education department or wellness center. Try these:

- Create a walking, riding, or running path around parts of campus that you usually do not get to see.
- Take an exercise class for credit.

- Join an intramural team.
- Ride your bike or walk to campus.
- Leave for class ten minutes earlier and walk a longer distance to your classes.

If you prefer to do your exercising at home, try some of these low-cost ideas.

Weightlifting
Create an inexpensive set of hand weights using empty milk jugs or dishwasher detergent bottles. Fill them with water or sand and secure the top with duct tape. By adding more water or sand to the jug, you can adjust the amount of weight as your fitness level changes.

Jump rope
Motivate yourself by jumping rope while watching your favorite TV show.

Strength training
Resistance tubing and bands are lightweight bands that come in different resistance levels. You can change the level of resistance by changing the way you hold the band. You can do both upper- and lower-body exercises with resistance bands.

Exercise videos
Create the feel of an aerobics class in your own room. Check out tapes from the library to get an idea of which instructors and what types of tapes you like the most, then pick a tape that matches your current fitness level.

Exercise for Every Season
The key to a lifetime of fitness is consistency. Here are some tips to help you make exercise a habit:

- Choose activities you like doing.
- Start your exercise pace at a level that matches your fitness (in both frequency and intensity), and increase from there.
- Set realistic goals.
- It takes time for our bodies to adjust to new routines. Don't be discouraged if you do not see results right away.
- If you miss a day of planned exercise, don't give up. Simply get back on track the next day.

- Schedule rest days into your exercise schedule.

- Listen to your body. If you have difficulty breathing or experience faintness or prolonged weakness during or after exercise, stop and consult your physician.

It's a good idea to choose more than one type of exercise to give your body a thorough workout and to prevent boredom. Choose one indoor exercise and one outdoor activity to allow for changes in your schedule or for inclement weather.

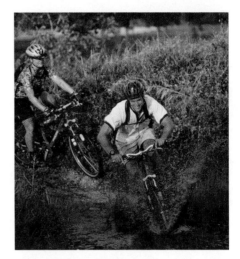

Exercising with other people will increase your motivation and enjoyment.

Lessons Learned from the Sumo Wrestlers

Sumo wrestlers are experts at putting on fat, which means the lessons they've learned can help us achieve a healthy body weight. If you do not want to gain pounds, follow these steps. The wrestlers, of course, will be doing just the opposite.

1. Eat small meals and snacks throughout the day.

2. Don't skip breakfast.

3. Never starve yourself.

4. Include fruits and vegetables with every meal.

5. Make food choices that honor your health and taste buds.

6. Watch your appetite when dining with family and friends.

7. Make your workouts slow and steady, not fast and frantic.

7

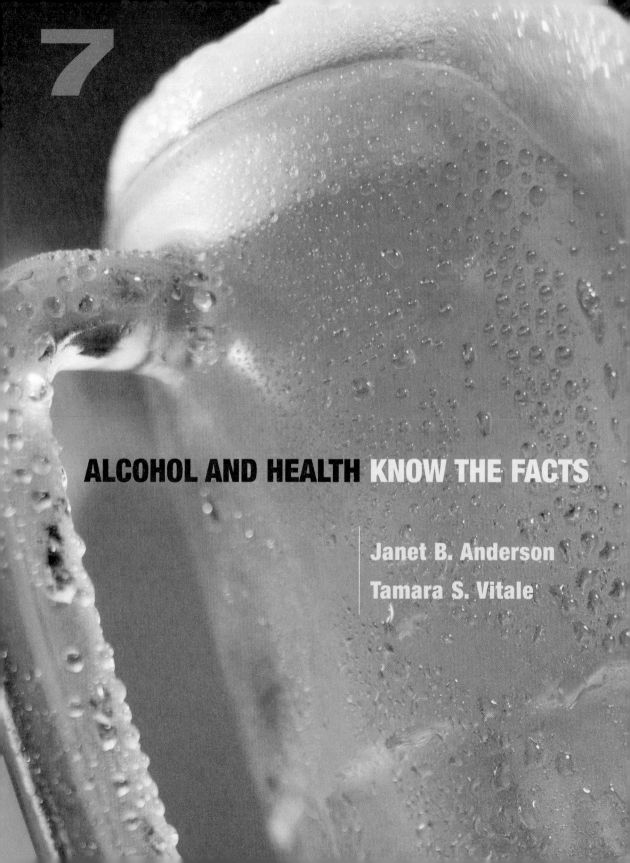

ALCOHOL AND HEALTH KNOW THE FACTS

Janet B. Anderson

Tamara S. Vitale

The decision of whether or not to drink is a personal choice. According to the 2005 Dietary Guidelines for Americans, 55% of U.S. adults consume alcohol, while 45% of U.S. adults do not drink any alcohol at all. Alcohol can have negative effects—it is highly addictive and can damage your body, diminish your self control, and increase your risk of injury and death. Despite this, alcohol is an important part of many college students' social life. The following questions and answers about alcohol and alcohol use will help you decide whether alcohol consumption will be a part of your healthy lifestyle.

Alcohol Questions and Answers

What are the laws and school policies I need to know?

Most universities and colleges have a very strict alcohol policy. For example, some schools have policies that prohibit possession, consumption, or distribution of alcoholic beverages on campus, including athletic events. Others have specific guidelines about how alcohol can be distributed. Most universities have their policy listed on the Web site. It's likely that you also received this information during your freshman orientation. If you live on campus, you can ask the resident advisor in your dorm if you are unclear about any policies.

It is illegal to buy or possess alcohol if you are under twenty-one. In some states, people under the age of twenty-one who are found to have any amount of alcohol in their systems can lose their driver's license, be subject to a heavy fine, or have their car permanently taken away. Drinking and driving is extremely dangerous. Whether you feel impaired or not, just one drink can make you fail a breath test.

What are the risks and dangers of alcohol use?

Binge drinking and drinking contests can result in physical and social problems, legal consequences, and even death. *Binge drinking* is defined as having five or more drinks on one occasion for males and three or more drinks at one sitting for females. About 15% of teens are binge drinkers in any given month, and college students in the 18–21-year-old range are most likely to engage in this behavior. Binge drinking is associated with higher rates of property damage, trouble with the law, poor class attendance, and injuries. Students living on campuses with high rates of binge drinking experience more incidents of assault and rape than students on campuses with lower binge drinking rates.

Binge drinking and drinking contests can cause a person to *black out,* or become unconscious. Immediate medical attention is necessary if a person becomes unconscious, is impossible to arouse, or seems to have trouble breathing. Drinking a high concentration of alcohol in a short period of time can suppress the centers of the brain that control breathing and cause a person to pass out or even die. When people pass out, their bodies continue to absorb alcohol. The amount of alcohol in the blood can reach dangerous levels, and they can die in their sleep. Continue to check on someone who has gone to sleep drunk. Do not leave that person alone.

Mixing alcohol with medications or illicit drugs is extremely dangerous and can lead to accidental death. Alcohol-medication interactions may be a factor in at least 25% of emergency room admissions. Check with your pharmacist about possible interactions if you are taking any prescription or over-the-counter medications and plan to use alcohol. Diabetics need to be especially cautious about drinking on an empty stomach, which can cause severe hypoglycemia.

How much alcohol do different drinks contain?

Alcohol content is given as a percentage. White wines average 12%, and red wines are around 14%. The alcohol content of beer is between 3% and 8%. "Light" or lower-calorie beers have fewer calories and are closer to 3% alcohol content. Liquor has the highest alcohol content, usually between 35% and 50%.

Proof is the percentage of alcohol (by volume) multiplied by two. For example:

100-proof alcohol = 50% alcohol
200-proof alcohol = 100% alcohol

Liqueurs, such as sherry and dessert liqueurs, contain 40 to 50% alcohol and tend to be higher in calories since they are sweetened.

What is "moderate" alcohol consumption?

The definition of moderate drinking is two drinks per day for men, and one for women and older people. A "drink" is defined as follows:

- One 12 oz. beer or wine cooler
- One 5 oz. glass of wine
- 1.5 ounces of 80-proof distilled spirits (a shotglass)

How do I know if I am drinking too much?

Alcohol is highly addictive. People under forty-five years old have higher rates of alcohol problems than do older people. Thirteen percent of male and 5% of female college students nationwide are alcoholic. Alcoholism tends to run in families.

The following signs can help you recognize if you are drinking too much:

- You feel you should cut down on your drinking.

- Others have criticized you for your drinking.

- You feel bad, guilty, or remorseful after drinking.

- You are not able to stop drinking once you have started.

- You fail to do what is normally expected from you because of drinking.

- You need a first drink in the morning to get yourself going after a heavy drinking session.

- You're unable to remember what happened the night before because you were drinking.

- You are injured as a result of your drinking.

- A relative, friend, or doctor expresses concern about your drinking or suggests that you cut down.

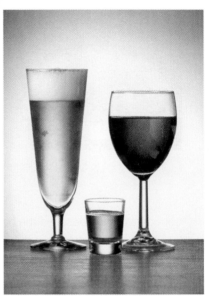

Each of these drinks contains the same amount of alcohol.

What causes a hangover?

Consuming too much alcohol can lead to a hangover. More than 75% of alcohol consumers have experienced a hangover at least once, 15% have one at least every month, and 25% of college students feel symptoms weekly. Some of the most common hangover symptoms are thirst, fatigue, nausea, vomiting, diarrhea, headache, lack of appetite, and a general sense of illness.

The main cause of the symptoms of a hangover is dehydration. Dehydration occurs because the alcohol acts on the brain to block the creation of a chemical that causes the body to lose more water through the kidneys. This is why drinkers have to make frequent trips to the bathroom after drinking alcohol and have an extremely dry mouth the morning after heavy drinking. Headaches result

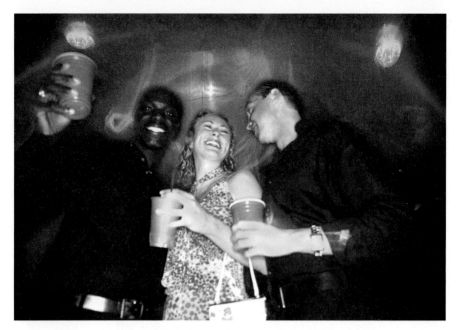
It's important to know your limits if you choose to drink alcohol.

from dehydration because the body's organs try to make up for their own water loss by stealing water from the brain. This causes the brain to decrease in size and pull on the membranes that connect the brain to the skull, resulting in pain. The frequent urination also expels sodium and potassium that are necessary for proper nerve and muscle function. This contributes to the headache, fatigue, and nausea.

Different types of alcohol can cause different types of hangover. This is because some types of alcoholic drink have a higher concentration of congeners, by-products of fermentation in some alcohol. Red wine, bourbon, brandy, cognac, tequila, and whiskey contain the greatest amounts of congeners, which are more likely to cause hangovers than other alcoholic beverages. White wine, rum, vodka, and gin have fewer congeners and therefore cause less frequent and less severe hangovers.

After a night of alcohol consumption, a drinker will not sleep as soundly as normal because the body is trying to rebound from alcohol's depressive effect on the system. Alcohol inhibits some of the body's natural stimulants, which makes you feel tired.

As you can see, taking a test or competing in an athletic event with a hangover isn't a great idea for many reasons.

What is the best hangover remedy?

The only foolproof way to avoid a hangover is not to drink alcohol, and the only cure for a hangover is time. No matter what you do, your body still has to clean up all of the toxic by-products left over from the alcohol, so your best bet is to not drink excessively in the first place.

The following general guidelines can help minimize the symptoms of a hangover:

Before drinking

- Eat a full meal. A full stomach slows down the absorption of alcohol and gives the body more time to process the toxins. A meal high in fat will increase this effect. Having food in the stomach also decreases stomach irritation.

- Drink a glass of water. This ensures the body is hydrated before the diuretic effect takes hold.

While drinking

- Drink in moderation. Ideally, drinkers should limit themselves to one drink per hour because the body takes about an hour to process a single drink.

- Drink a glass of water after every alcoholic beverage. In addition to helping keep a drinker hydrated, this will give the body more time to process the alcohol, dilute the toxins, and reduce irritation of the stomach. A sports drink will also replenish electrolytes, salts, and sugars lost in the urine while drinking.

- Watch your drink choice. Drinkers generally fare better when they stick with one drink. Each new type of alcohol makes the body work that much harder and puts that many more toxins in the body, leading to a more severe hangover.

- The effects of alcohol are accentuated in the heat, such as at the beach and in the hot tub. These conditions contribute to dehydration, which increases the effects of alcohol and is more likely to result in a hangover.

After drinking

- Take two aspirin with a full glass of water before going to bed. This can decrease hangover severity.

- Take two more aspirin with a full glass of water in the morning. This will help minimize headaches as well as decrease inflammation.

continued

- Eat breakfast. A meal that includes eggs (for the cysteine), a banana (for the potassium), and fruit juice (for the fructose) or a sports drink (for the electrolytes, sugars, and salts) can get the body on the road to recovery. Keep in mind that caffeinated coffee, tea, and soda will further dehydrate someone with a hangover.

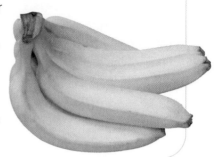

What effect does drinking have on my nutritional status?

Alcohol is not a food. It does not meet any dietary needs and in fact impairs the absorption of essential nutrients because it can damage the lining of the small intestine and the stomach where most nutrients are digested.

Alcoholic beverages supply calories but few nutrients, such as vitamins and minerals. As a result, excessive alcohol consumption makes it difficult to ingest sufficient nutrients within an individual's daily calorie allotment and to maintain a healthy weight. Although the consumption of one to two alcoholic beverages per day is not associated with nutrient deficiencies or with overall dietary quality, heavy drinkers may be at risk of malnutrition if the calories derived from alcohol are substituted for those in nutritious foods.

What can I learn from labels on alcoholic beverages?

Ever wonder how many calories, carbohydrates, or cholesterol might be in your favorite alcoholic beverage? The labels don't provide this information, although it is required on other food and beverage containers. Current labeling rules are a patchwork of antiquated federal requirements, each different for beer, wine, and spirits. For example, beer does not have to list alcohol content, but wine and distilled spirits with more than 14% alcohol do.

The only consistent notice on all alcoholic beverages is a warning about the health consequences of alcohol consumption. There is no standard serving size that tells consumers how many drinks are in a bottle, nor any requirement for ingredient or nutrition labeling. (There are regulations if a label makes dietary claims such as describing a beverage as "lite.")

How can I prevent weight gain while still including moderate alcohol in my diet?

The calories in alcohol can easily add up. Young drinkers often order fancy cocktails and don't realize how high in calories they are (see Table 7.1).

People who drink moderately tend to consume alcohol calories on top of their regular caloric intake. These excess calories promote body fat accumulation, particularly in the trunk area—the well-known "spare tire." The bottom line is that it's harder to feel full when alcohol becomes a part of your diet because alcohol stimulates the appetite. To maintain a lean machine, abstain or choose drinks that are lowest in calories.

Will alcohol affect my athletic performance?

Alcohol and athletics do not mix well. You can't be sharp, quick, and drunk. Alcohol has a negative effect on reaction time, accuracy, balance, eye-hand coordination, and endurance. It is a poor source of carbohydrates, which is the primary fuel source for athletes. Beer, instead of water, is often a significant source of postexercise fluids. Yet the alcohol in beer has a diuretic effect—the more you drink, the more fluids you lose. This is bad for recovery and often bad for the next exercise bout. While low-alcohol beer allows for proper rehydration, regular beer sends athletes running to the bathroom. One study showed that athletes who drank beer eliminated about 16 ounces more urine (over the course of four hours) than those who drank low-alcohol (2%) beer or alcohol-free beer (Shirreffs and Maughan 1997).

Exercise does not increase alcohol metabolism. After a hard workout, alcohol on an empty stomach can quickly contribute to a drunken stupor. Late-night partying contributes to getting too little sleep. This can create problems with next-morning events. For optimal performance, minimize alcohol intake.

How can I say no to alcohol and still fit in?

You do not have to drink when other people drink or because a drink is given to you. This is a personal decision each time you find yourself in a situation where alcohol is available. Make this decision based on your own knowledge, experiences, and desires. Remember that the majority of students do not drink alcohol. Practice ways to say no politely.

- If you choose to abstain, make up your mind to say no before you are ever in the situation.
- Tell people that you feel better when you drink less.

- Stay away from people who give you a hard time about not drinking.
- Learn to hold a glass or beer bottle for a long time, and refill it with whatever you want (such as water or club soda).

Table 7.1 How Many Calories Are in That Drink?

Beverage	Serving Volume	Approximate Total Calories
Beer (regular)	12 oz.	144
Beer (light)	12 oz.	108
White wine	5 oz.	100
Red wine	5 oz.	105
Sweet dessert wine	3 oz.	141
Margarita (2 oz. tequila, 2 oz. margarita/sour mix, 1 oz. triple sec, lime juice, and 1 tsp. sugar)	5 oz.	550
Long Island iced tea (1 oz. each vodka, gin, rum, tequila, and triple sec; 2 oz. sour mix; and a splash of soda)	7 oz.	380
White Russian (1.5 oz. vodka, 1.5 oz. coffee liqueur, and 1.5 oz. cream)	4.5 oz.	320
Piña colada (1.5 oz. rum, 1.5 oz. coconut cream, and 3 oz. pineapple juice)	6 oz.	293
Rum and Diet Coke (1 oz. rum)	7 oz.	65
Vodka and soda (1 oz. vodka)	7 oz.	65

continued

Beverage	Serving Volume	Approximate Total Calories
White wine spritzer (4 oz. white wine topped with club soda)	5 oz.	80
Bloody Mary (1 oz. vodka, 4 oz. tomato juice, and dash of Tabasco and pepper)	5 oz.	90

General Tips for Safe Alcohol Use

- Never drink just for the sake of drinking, as a game or contest, or with the aim of getting drunk or forgetting troubles.

- Determine how many drinks you will set as your limit, and stick to it.

- Communicate your limits—Practice techniques that you will use to communicate your limit. Know when to say, "Enough." Monitor your own feelings. Be wary of any changes in mood or perceptions.

- Utilize a buddy system—Make sure that you have a friend who will stick with you and keep you safe. This is especially important as sexual inhibitions are reduced with alcohol consumption. After all, you wouldn't want to wake up in someone's bed and wonder how you got there. This happens—sad, but true.

- Mix your own drinks or know who is mixing them. Be wary of date-rape drugs.

- Designate a driver—Have someone designated to drive if you're going to drink, or plan an alternative way home, such as a taxi or bus.

- Know the warning signs of drinking too much—After drinking, people usually feel pleasure and become happy, talkative, and boastful at first. The feelings are usually replaced by drowsiness as the alcohol is eliminated from the body, and the drinker may become withdrawn. This pattern often encourages people to drink more to keep the buzz going. Continued drinking leads to a staggering gait, crying spells, slurred speech, nausea, and vomiting.

- Do not drink on an empty stomach. Snack before and during alcohol use.

- When you drink, sip your drink slowly. Take a one-hour break between drinks. Drink soda, water, or juice after a drink with alcohol.

- Drink a large glass of water before going to bed.

- Do not take any medication with alcohol without checking with your pharmacist or doctor.

89

References

Cho, S., M. Dietrich, C. J. P. Brown, C. A. Clark, and G. Bloc. 2003. The effect of breakfast type on total daily energy intake and body mass index: results from the third national health and nutrition examination survey (NHANES III). *Journal of the American College of Nutrition* 22: 296–302.

Ginsberg, C., and A. Ostrowski. 2002. The market for vegetarian foods. *Vegetarian Journal* 4: 25–29.

Mokdad, A. H., J. S. Marks, D. F. Stroup, and J. L. Gerberding. 2004. Actual causes of death in the United States, 2000. *Journal of the American Medical Association* 291: 1238–45.

National Center for Health Statistics. 2004. Prevalence of overweight and obesity among adults: United States, 1999–2002. www.cdc.gov/nchs/products/pubs/pubd/hestats/obese/obse99.htm.

Shirreffs, S. M., and R. J. Maughan. 1997. Restoration of fluid balance after exercise-induced dehydration: effects of alcohol consumption. *Journal of Applied Physiology* 83: 1152–58.

Vegetarian Resource Group. 2000. How many vegetarians are there? www.vrg.org/nutshell/poll2000.htm.

Wing, R., and S. Phelan. 2005. Long-term weight loss maintenance. *American Journal of Clinical Nutrition* 82 (1): 222S–25S.

EAT RIGHT! HEALTHY EATING IN COLLEGE AND BEYOND